T0303881

Frightful Stages:
From the Primitive
to the Therapeutic

Robert B. Marchesani
E. Mark Stern
Editors

Frightful Stages: From the Primitive to the Therapeutic has been co-published simultaneously as *The Psychotherapy Patient*, Volume 11, Numbers 3/4 2001.

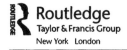

Routledge
Taylor & Francis Group
New York   London

Routledge is an imprint of the
Taylor & Francis Group, an informa business

Frightful Stages: From the Primitive to the Therapeutic has been co-published simultaneously as *The Psychotherapy Patient*, Volume 11, Numbers 3/4 2001.

Reprinted 2009 by Routledge

The development, preparation, and publication of this work has been undertaken with great care. However, the publisher, employees, editors, and agents of The Haworth Press and all imprints of The Haworth Press, Inc., including The Haworth Medical Press® and Pharmaceutical Products Press®, are not responsible for any errors contained herein or for consequences that may ensue from use of materials or information contained in this work. Opinions expressed by the author(s) are not necessarily those of The Haworth Press, Inc.

Cover design by Thomas J. Mayshock Jr.

Cover photo: From the collection of Carl Van Vechten's works at the United States Library of Congress. Used by permission.

Photo of Robert B. Marchesani by Antonio Gabriel.

Library of Congress Cataloging-in-Publication Data

Frightful stages : from the primitive to the therapeutic / Robert B. Marchesani, E. Mark Stern, editors.
     p. cm.
     "Has been co-published simultaneously as the Psychotherapy patient, volume 11, numbers 3/4 2001."
     Includes bibliographical references and index.
     ISBN 0-7890-1365-7 (alk. paper)–ISBN 0-7890-1366-5 (alk. paper)
     1. Psychotherapy. 2. Awe. 3. Existential psychology. 4. Experiential psychotherapy. I. Marchesani, Robert B. II. Stern, E. Mark, 1929-
RC480.5 .F7554 2001
616.89'14–dc21   2001024215

Frightful Stages:
From the Primitive to the Therapeutic

CONTENTS

ABOUT THE EDITORS

Robert B. Marchesani, MSS, is a psychotherapist in private practice in New York and Philadelphia. Mr. Marchesani is co-editor of *The Psychotherapy Patient* and holds a degree in Psychoanalytic Studies from New School University in New York. He currently is a senior candidate at The Philadelphia School of Psychoanalysis and teaches "The Internet and the Hyper-Self" in The New School's cyberspace program (www.dialnsa. edu).

E. Mark Stern, EdD, ABPP, is a Fellow of the American Psychological Association, the American Psychological Society, and the Academy of Clinical Psychology. Dr. Stern is Emeritus Professor, Graduate School of Arts and Sciences at Iona College in New Rochelle, New York. He has taught at Seton Hall University, Fordham University, and Catholic University of Australia, and he has lectured and made professional presentations throughout the United States, Canada, and Great Britain. Dr. Stern has been president of two divisions of the American Psychological Association, the Division of the Psychology of Religion (received the Mentoring Award) and the Division of Humanistic Psychology (awarded the Carl Rogers Award). He has served four terms on the Council of Representatives, which is the governing board of The American Psychological Association. Dr. Stern has been the Editor of *The Journal of Pastoral Counseling* and *VOICES: The Journal of the American Academy of Psychotherapy*. He is currently the Editor of *The Psychotherapy Patient Series* and Senior Editor (Psychotherapy) of The Haworth Press, Inc.

Awe: Dionysian and Apollonian
(A Preface)

Awe raises the possibilities of passion. Those awed may be ambushed by inescapable longings. But they may be the high priests of idols, plagued by the demands of the golden calf. Their dreams of adoration submerge into preoccupation. They are servants of adored icons.

The Hebrew Bible condemns the followers of Abraham who become enraptured by the false faces of Molech. Idolizing awe ends the culture of dialogue; no colloquy in the presence of idol worship.

Awe cannot be limited to a single leitmotif. Saint Augustine was aware of the encroaching compulsion to grip at the ephemeral. Faith in its presence as awe holds dear those mysteries that rendered the true god of true gods before the day of creation.

Awe is a unique complexity, trembling not only with the unbridled sensations of Dionysius, but also into the lurking prospects of Apollo. Dionysian awe penetrates into the frenzy of the frustrated community. A Mozart or a Hitler could result. Apollonian consciousness, while acting in accord with the community, awakens the unsuspecting slumberer to the astonishment of his or her unknown potentialities.

So it was that a fabled Job-like Jew, not as yet touched by Apollo, suffered the demise of his family and wealth in a small *shetl* (community) in Eastern Europe. The turn of the nineteenth century was still some decades in the future. The man's daughter died in childbirth; his son vanished in a faraway expedition and his wife suddenly became feeble and finally expired. Tormented beyond belief, the man's counting house ended in ruin. His generosity and his being held in reverent esteem survived.

The man's privations were not lost on the community. The Days of Awe were upon them–ten days of prayerful interval between the Jewish New Year and the Day of Atonement–days in which one asks much the same forgiveness of one's neighbor that one is about to ask of God.

[Haworth co-indexing entry note]: "Awe: Dionysian and Apollonian (A Preface)." Stern, E. Mark. Co-published simultaneously in *The Psychotherapy Patient* (The Haworth Press, Inc.) Vol. 11, No. 3/4, 2001, pp. xvii-xviii; and: *Frightful Stages: From the Primitive to the Therapeutic* (ed: Robert B. Marchesani, and E. Mark Stern) The Haworth Press, Inc., 2001, pp. xiii-xiv. Single or multiple copies of this article are available for a fee from The Haworth Document Delivery Service [1-800-342-9678, 9:00 a.m. - 5:00 p.m. (EST). E-mail address: getinfo@haworthpressinc.com].

The community too was short on resources. There was no cantor to chant the holy words of intercession. And without an intercessor there is danger that opportunistic idols dressed as demons might descend into their midst. Dionysian murmurs were everywhere to be heard. Perhaps it would be best to embrace the demons; forgo the ritual penitence; dance the dance of the chaotic.

Still the man was where he was in his life in the village. The senior counselors conferred. Apollonic reason quartered with Dionysian inspiration. The man would receive their ordination as Cantor. Protesting that he had no voice for such a high calling, for the Days of Awe, the elders consulted with a neighboring rabbi since the community had no means of supporting a rabbi of its own. The rabbi took due note of the man's torments and doubts. But it was above all that the man's stutters and trembles of which he took particular note. Trembling and verbal falters were the keynotes of Moses' calling: "This man is beyond privation. He is well-prepared to cast away worldly illusions." This awe alone is denoted by the Kabbalah as *rasha d'la yad 'a ud' ityad'a* (the all knowing source that remains free of ever being discerned).

Psychotherapists who, in this day, cease to be "knowing" approach the shifting deployments of awe in stunned humility. On behalf of the individual within the community, psychotherapists remain humbly mystified by how people hold sacred the Dionysian and Apollonian in their experiences. For a client to be flooded with the ambitions of a seductive culture; for a client to be overtaken by fears of the morning, the afternoon, the evening, the night; for a client to not want to be; for a client to want to be exempted from ever being beheld; for a client needing to move in directions never before explored . . .

It is the hope of the editors of this volume that awe will further sensitize its readers to seductions and powers beyond mere scrutiny.

E. Mark Stern
The Psychotherapy Patient *Series Editor*

Introduction–
A Hermit in Times Square:
Setting the Stage

Rob Marchesani

When he has exhausted all avenues and methods of creativeness an actor reaches a limit beyond which human consciousness cannot extend. Here begins the realm of the unconscious, of intuition, which is not accessible to mind but is to feelings, not to thought but to creative emotions. An actor's unpolished technique cannot reach it; it is accessible only to his artist-nature.

Unfortunately, the realm of the unconscious is often ignored in our art because most actors limit themselves to superficial feelings, and the spectators are satisfied with purely external impressions. Yet the essence of art and the main source of creativeness are hidden deep in man's soul; there, in the center of our spiritual being, in the realm of our inaccessible superconsciousness, our mysterious 'I' has its being, and inspiration itself. That is the storehouse of our most important spiritual material.

–Stanislavski/*Creating a Role*

In a treatise on free association and self-analysis, Karen Horney wrote: "... it is essential to abstain from reasoning while associating" (1942). I discovered this one particularly sultry night while unable to get offline from a late-night Internet excursion one summer. Having had bouts of curiosity with the many unknown others at the ends of the Internet galaxy, I went on a quest, all the while holding in fantasy the suitor I was seeking.

[Haworth co-indexing entry note]: "Introduction–A Hermit in Times Square: Setting the Stage." Marchesani, Rob. Co-published simultaneously in *The Psychotherapy Patient* (The Haworth Press, Inc.) Vol. 11, No. 3/4, 2001, pp. 1-9; and: *Frightful Stages: From the Primitive to the Therapeutic* (ed: Robert B. Marchesani, and E. Mark Stern) The Haworth Press, Inc., 2001, pp. 1-9. Single or multiple copies of this article are available for a fee from The Haworth Document Delivery Service [1-800-342-9678, 9:00 a.m. - 5:00 p.m. (EST). E-mail address: getinfo@haworthpressinc.com].

It was a strange moment, a breakthrough of sorts, when my hands left the keyboard and I turned to my library behind me. There, Horney's book *Self-Analysis* pointed itself out to my attention. It goes without saying just what this mysterious phenomenon is about–the turning of one's attention to some-thing else while in the midst of a completely different task only to find exactly what one needs to know at the moment. It happened to Augustine of Hippo once, only by divine intervention, when he was prompted to take and read The Good Book. Opening it at random his eyes fell upon the precise passage he needed to read to find the meaning of a crucial turning point in his life. Something said, "tole lege," and he took and read. . . .

I began to wonder about spontaneity and the creation of art. And also of the inhibitions to spontaneity. About a year prior, in another unusual find, this time in a little shop of odd trinkets and other seemingly ordinary objects, there in the middle of the floor was a pile of small shiny bright orange books: *The Essential Salvador Dali* by Robert Goff (1998). "Freud's theories on dreams have such an immense influence on the impressionable Dali that they change forever the essentials of his art. Dali's interests and energies, from this point onward, become channeled through the lens of Freudian psychoanalytic theory" (p. 26). Besides his great works of art, Dali created a way of working with the productions of artists, particularly the Surrealists who relied on automatic writing and free association. With Freud's insights, Dali ap-proached Surrealism with what he termed the paranoiac-critical method. The paranoia, the unconscious dream material, Dali believed, needed to be orga-nized consciously, intellectually, critically. For Dali, it wasn't enough to rely on "psychic automatism" which Andre Breton described, nor on chance effects–the way of expressing the unconscious for the Surrealists–a way that Dali believed to be inefficient. According to Goff, "His approach gives artists a method for organizing their own obsessions and presenting them on the canvas in a way that helps them know themselves better." The whole point of free association–to know one's deepest thoughts. Back to Horney. And perhaps even to Freud.

The method of interpretation was Freud's attempt to organize the material he uncovered along the royal road of our dreams, his own included. Freud's journey with patients began like the journey to Oz–with Dorothy's dream of the tornado, an apt metaphor for the wildness of the unconscious, a vortex connecting the underworld with the overworld, if you will, of the psyche. The dream also ties the story together, connecting dream personas with the real-life personalities in Dorothy's life. Without the dream, there would be no story. Without a personal story, there would be no psychotherapy.

While Mark Stern and I were working on *Awe and Trembling* (co-pub-lished as *The Psychotherapy Patient* 11([1/2]), Tobi Zausner had thoroughly captured my attention in the world of Edvard Munch. Like Dali's paranoia,

Munch's art showed an emphasis on fright–consider *Scream* and *Anxiety*. And consider too how audiences have focused so much on the experience of fright, no doubt significant in their own lives, and one begins to feel that the audience and the artist are entering a similar space, albeit for one it is a space of exhibition, for the other a space of private musings. The audience, then, becomes the listener–the observer of the product of the artist's own observations, the artist's own attentiveness. The demand of the unconscious in the artist: to exhibit. The drive in the audience: to look and to hear. And in both there is often something to feel. The Italian verb *sentire* means both *to listen to* and *to feel*. It may be that art, theater and other productions perk up our ears, as well as our emotions, to that which lies dormant–unmoved by what we just might pass each day, or by what passes us. When we listen, we begin to feel. And when we feel, we just might begin to listen.

What Goff attributes to Dali, which we may also acknowledge as Freud's contribution to Dali and to art, is a grappling with the question, "What to do with this impulse?" Ah, first you must have the impulse to know what it is, Horney might say. Let us lie back and let ourselves be for a moment. Is this not what the Internet has allowed us to do on many a late night? But the intrusion of one's conscience interferes. Superego stands ready to shake its head in disapproval, looking down on us, ready to make its attack. What if we let ourselves go, for a moment, in this new free space? What if we let the words flow without critique, without judgment, then sit back and look at what came out? Then, analyze the data we have collected or simply the experience we've had? Isn't that the stuff of research, regardless of the subject matter? As Aristotle knew, research begins with wonder. And wonder is at the beginning of many a desire to perform and to create. Consider actors who research characters for their roles, letting themselves be different, an act which often changes their body and appearance, challenging body egos and demanding something more. Something different.

We sit with patients who sit with themselves each day and night until they meet with us. We may wonder what it is that makes this person's life meaningful (and what obstructs it). What it is that constitutes a person's experience (and what diminishes it). These words are not easy to write for an audience as diverse and divergent as the one known as psychotherapists, as well as those who have experienced various forms of this wide field. They, you–*we* comprise psychiatrists, psychoanalysts, psychologists, social workers, and a host of others from various fields, and within each, the divisions of practice and approach continue. Yet, whether taking medication for anxiety, whether channeling behavior away from destructive impulses, whether examining unconscious motivations and personal constructions, we stand on a fine line between knowing and not knowing what it is that is creative and enlivening for each person, for each of us. In his writing on Hans Loewald, Lawrence

Friedman (*On the Therapeutic Action of Loewald's Theory*, 1991) may have captured what therapists of any persuasion must provide:

> Loewald has solved a central mystery of all talking treatments: Quite apart from what the analyst does by his interpretations, patients treat themselves by talking *to* an interpreter, that is, by trying to make themselves known to someone they assume can interpret. Loewald tells us why the patient is helped by that very activity. The difference in levels of organization between patient and analyst belongs as much to the patient as to the analyst. By translating his unspoken mind into the language of an imagined understander, the patient is growing himself up. It is the reach and not just the grasp that does the work.

It seems that the project of psychotherapy is one that is constantly evolving in our work with patients and in our patients' work with themselves. That is why people like Karen Horney and, in this volume, Al Mahrer are advocates of self-analysis, or self-therapy, yet not without direction. When the late sociologist Benjamin Nelson wrote that "a new era in the history of spiritual direction begins with Freud" (*Self Images and Systems of Spiritual Direction* in *On the Roads to Modernity: Conscience, Science, and Civilizations* [1981 (1965)]), he was referring to the evolution of therapy. "Freud explains elsewhere that he was spurred on to develop psychoanalysis as a distinctive set of procedures in the hope of improving upon available methods of therapy, notably the electrotherapy of Erb, the relaxation therapy of Weir Mitchell and the rational therapy of Dubois (Freud 1914)" (Nelson, p. 57). But even the evolution of therapy may not be so linear and logical and so many of the therapies of the last century can be found today in various forms and with various adaptations. With so many approaches, we may finally get the long-known and often forgotten message, "There is nothing new under the sun." Yet, what is often searched for in treatment is some newness, something fresh and vibrant, and it is this experience that often drives people to the work of psychotherapy.

Since Freud's writing, we have turned many a new corner, but not without encountering many an old one, a familiar one, a human one. It was Alexander Smith's piece on Thomas Merton and Gregory Zilboorg that inspired the title for this introduction. Merton himself authored a small book, *Spiritual Direction and Meditation* (1960), as well as numerous other titles on spirituality. Smith gives us an account of Merton's encounters with the analyst Zilboorg (who contributed to one of Nelson's collections, *Freud and the 20th Century*). In that account, Smith reports what Zilboorg thought of the hermitage which Merton struggled to balance with his growing fame: "You want a hermitage in Times Square with a large sign over it saying HERMIT." Smith also points out that Merton was reading Horney and Jung. In a recently published book, *The Intimate Merton: His Life from His Journals* (1999), Merton writes: "Ever since I was sixteen traveling all over Europe, some of it on foot by myself (always by preference alone), I have developed this terrific sense of geography, this habit of self-analysis, this knack of getting along with strangers and chance acquaintances–this complete independence and self-dependence, which turns out to be not a strength but, in my big problem, a terrific weakness." Merton wrote that in 1941, just one year before Horney's book on self-analysis was published. In his essay, *The Concept of a Healthy Individual*, D. W. Winnicott expressed his thoughts about independence: "Individual maturity implies a movement towards independence, but there is no such thing as independence. It would be unhealthy for an individual to be so withdrawn as to feel independent and invulnerable. If such a person is alive, then there is dependence indeed!" (1986 [1967]).

Another passage from Merton's journals shows how much of a theater he was facing with Zilboorg and the Abbot and that there are other productions that lie in our midst besides the stage and screen:

> I thought today, what a blessing it was that I did not go in 1956 to be analyzed by Gregory Zilboorg! What a tragedy and mess that would have been–and I must give Z. the credit for having sensed it himself in his own way. It would have been utterly impossible and absurd. I think in great measure his judgment was that I could not be fitted into his kind of theater. There was no conceivable part for me to play in his life. . . . He had quite enough intelligence (more than enough, he was no fool at all!) to see that it would be a very poor production for him, for the Abbot (who was most willing), and for me. . . . In any case, all manner of better things were reserved for me. But I have not understood them.

Merton's "big problem" may have been his independence, but the fact that he ended his life in search of a bridge to the East to join its spirituality with the West may have taken another turn had Merton made such a bridge right here in the West by doing just what Zilboorg recognized, had he taken a different tone with Merton. A hermitage sporting the sign HERMIT might just have been what Times Square, the center of Broadway Theater, needed and it may have been what the church needed. It could have been subtitled THE LISTENING BOOTH and attracted many to the wisdom of contemplation. Emerson knew the perfection of solitude was not in isolation but in the midst of a crowd and in no other place can a crowd be a crowd quite as it can be in Times Square. When it was announced on the eve of the millennium that some 2 million people converged in a twenty-block area around Times Square, I'd thought, "That's nearly the entire population of Philadelphia and its counties!" It was unimaginable to me, a transplant from Philadelphia to

Manhattan. But the Fates had other things in store for Merton. And for Times Square.

But as Smith shows, the drama created by the Abbot and the many collusive and complicating parties made it impossible for Merton to step onto the true analytic stage, the one that is more like one's visit to a spiritual director or confessor–without the interference of others, without anyone else but "I and Thou," which was foreclosed to Merton and Zilboorg.

Besides Merton and Zilboorg, two other accounts of public figures and their work have been prepared for us. Freud's analysis did not stop in the consulting room, nor was it limited to its quarters where Freud produced his analytic accounts of other figures he'd only encountered in art or other writings. Stern's account and analysis of Carl Van Vechten and Bessie Smith and Mendelowitz's writing on Fellini's *Nights of Cabiria* show us a few things about artists and their work. They also show us a thing or two about suffering and redemption. Stern and Mendelowitz have each given us a study of character in several media, not limited to the personal interview of the therapist's office, which each of these authors maintains. Stern presents an historical account not only of the lives of two American personages but also of the cultural life of America, New York, the art scene and the Renaissance of Harlem, all within the psychological framework of a biography rich in fine (and sometimes grim) detail, finally breaking the spell of the awestruck. Stern points our attention to the dangers of relationships in which each party holds the other in awe.

As much as the stage may lure many a starry-eyed performer in search of a spotlight, it may also paralyze the willing subject when least expected. The retreat will send the poor subject, along with his therapist, to hell and back as the trip through psychotherapy reconstructs the hidden dramas that trip one on the way to the spotlight, something which Isaac Tylim ("One Sings, the Other Doesn't: Stage Fright and the Psychoanalytic Theater") will illuminate for the singer who finds himself alone on the stage and, like Barbra Streisand ("From the Couch to *The Concert*: Streisand as Doctor and Patient"), unable to be there, for a time, until they've worked through the terrors that prevented them from returning to their respective stages. In yet another account, this time from the direct experience of an actor himself, Pietro Arpesella ("The Little Old Lady") will recount his own dealing with performance anxiety and give us something to think about concerning one's childhood disturbances and the psychological origins of diabetes.

It's what people have inside them that we wonder about. It's what they allow out and *how* they allow what's inside to come out that concerns us. In both psychotherapy and in theater, we find two things of continual fascination, interest, and engagement: what people are doing and what they are thinking. In this regard, the director and the therapist sit in the same chair of the contemplative. Edward Smith ("Awe and Terror in the Living of the Resolution of the Polarity of Insight and Expression") takes us on the tightrope of insight and expression using elements of psychodrama and psychoanalysis to land us on a firmer footing about such stages.

We've tried two new ways of interviewing this time. One makes use of e-mail, my conversation with Mark Stern, the other with a combination of Instant Messaging and e-mail, with Casey Fraser, a stand-up comic and improvisationist. While much of what we included contains themes of stage fright and other forms of performance anxiety, including the private kind that the poet experiences as John Schertzer will invite us to entertain, we go beyond. *Frightful Stages* is meant to connote not only the experiences of acting and performing but also those moments and times in life when something tells us a thing or two about our lives and the story that frightens us, cajoles us, and causes us to reconsider it and ourselves in the context of the world that we call ours. Kirk Schneider, David Elkins, L. M. Leitner and Al Mahrer concentrate their efforts on the dimensions of awe in psychotherapy. Their papers were presented at the American Psychological Association's annual meeting in 1999. Speaking of frightful stages, Charles Tart ("I'm Not Crazy, They Are Coming Around with Guns!") will take us on a journey of fear and the uncanny from his own personal experience, as will Scott Churchill ("On Anguish and Other Frightful Moments in the Process of Self-Discovery").

When I began writing this introduction, Augustine came to mind. Now that I am about to conclude it, he seems to return, this time in thinking about the importance of mothers and their relationships with their children in the formation of their character. Augustine's mother was relentless in her pursuit of her son's vocation. Like the church itself, often referred to then as the Holy Mother church, she chased after her son as though she'd had a greater investment in his vocation than he did, *until* he did. So mothers are on my mind. During a break from composing this introduction, I was on the phone with my own mother one evening. She asked what this next book was going to be about. Among other issues, stage fright, I said. You don't have to be on stage to have that, she said. She proceeded to tell me how difficult it can be just to talk to people. I told her that some people can be difficult to talk to. An excerpt from Schertzer's essay seems right to call upon: "Such a perspective makes one aware of the *performance anxiety* that goes on continually in life, in every aspect, since being human involves an unrelenting struggle of self-composition. The same drives which render one whole also serve to disrupt that wholeness; the forces modeling a 'self' also play a part in disintegrating it."

"Psychoanalysis seems to be more popular," Mother continued. "More and more people seem to need it." I was shocked to hear the good news. To my knowledge, I was the only one in my family who'd ever done it, as if psychoanalysis is only something to do. I'm beginning to think it's a way of being, or at least a way of thinking, a way of being attentive, and present. "Yes," she continued. "I heard on the radio the other day that it's helpful for many people." After such tragedies as Columbine High, I should think there would be a need for more such work toward the diffusion of aggression into words that could save lives.

When you edit a publication two great fears emerge. One, that what some people submit will not work well with what others submit. But since we have two issues in this volume, forgive us our departures from the topic at hand. Rather, take this collection as a view of stage fright and other terrors from *in front of* and from *behind* the curtain that separates our public lives from our private lives. Consider, too, the old saying "all the world's a stage," and suddenly–whether in a theater, at a dinner party, whether one on one behind closed doors or alone online–the distinctions begin to blur.

During yet another break, this time while gardening in the nearby J. J. Walker Park in Greenwich Village, I wondered whether I should be there or at my desk working on further revisions. Something said, I imagined, shift the process from your head to your hands–knock yourself out! As I was pulling out a handful of weeds, I heard a voice from behind. A friend I hadn't seen in a while said, "You know I planted those last year." My heart thumped and I remembered his humor. "These?" I asked, looking into his knowing eyes. It was Les Lone, a semi-retired filmmaker. He asked about the progress of the book. I told him where I was. He said, Sir Lawrence Olivier used to take time before each performance and stand behind the curtain. "He'd look through a peep hole cursing the audience. For 15 minutes he would do this because he so feared the audience. That's how he dealt with his stage fright. It sort of calmed his nerves. It was his way of saying to them, *I love you all for coming but you're scaring the crap out of me.*" According to Les, this is why many famous Hollywood actors do not return to Broadway Theater. "There's no audience to perform for in making movies. There's only the actor and the camera along with the director and the crew. If the actor wants to do another take the director will usually cooperate." Ensemble acting forms a protection which the solo actor does not have. Such an actor has the group to help. Which might explain the prevalence of stage fright among those who go it alone. But my conversation with Les went further to include other forms of stage fright. Having been deemed the number-one fear of Americans, public speaking is another form that might also be seen among other professions. Les explained, "Out of a thousand attorneys who graduate, for instance, only a small percentage are litigators, those who plead your case before a jury." Another stage.

The other fear in editing a publication is writing the introduction. What to write about, how to say it, and how to introduce what follows. Deadline anxiety may be another form of performance anxiety. The best remedy for writer's block may be simply to write. To engage a free-writing, a free association on the page which is a way of letting what's inside come out. Like improvisation–using the material at hand to create something new. Something we practice everyday with our patients or clients (I like neither word myself) and something that everyday beckons us to attempt to refine in our own lives, except that in therapy, we ask that the editing function be turned off while we find out what's so difficult to say. But revisions will come as part of our productions. The critical faculties will follow the irrational.

I'll leave the last word of this introduction for another writer who manages to address stage fright, writer's block and perhaps even the most important benefit of psychotherapy:

> For I believe the greatest cause of writer's block, not to mention stage fright, is the fear that one has nothing to say–not that one doesn't know how to say it. . . . It (writing) is a way of thinking, a way of looking at the world, and a way of processing information that not only contributes to stories, articles, and books but also enhances one's appreciation of life. (Stewart, 1999)

REFERENCES

Friedman, L. (1991). On the therapeutic action of Loewald's theory. In Fogel, G. (Ed.), The work of Hans Loewald. New Jersey, London: Jason Aronson Inc.

Horney, K. (1942). Self-analysis. New York, London: WW Norton and Company.

Goff, R. (1998). The essential Salvador Dali. New York: The Wonderland Press.

Lone, L. (2000). Private communication. New York.

Merton, T. (1999). Montaldo, J. and Hart, P. (Eds.). The Intimate Merton: his life from his journals. San Francisco: Harper.

Nelson, B. (1965). Self-images and systems of spiritual direction. In Huff, Toby E. (Ed.) (1981), On the roads to modernity: conscience, science, and civilizations. Totowa, New Jersey: Rowman and Littlefield.

Stanislavski, C. (1961). Creating a role. New York: Routledge.

Stewart, J. (1999). The authors guild bulletin.

Winnicott, D. W. (1967). The concept of a healthy individual. In (1986) Home is where we start from: essays by a psychoanalyst. New York and London: WW Norton and Company.

One Sings, the Other Doesn't:
Stage Fright and the Psychoanalytic Theater

Isaac Tylim

SUMMARY. This paper attempts to explore the psychodynamics of stage fright, elucidating the differences between stage fright and social phobia. Special attention is paid to stage fright as a significant symptom of performers. The function of stage fright in impeding or benefiting performance is also addressed. Performers' affective states will be contrasted to impostors' and their psychological dimensions will be studied. The vicissitudes of the psychoanalytic treatment of a performer who suffered from severe stage fright will illustrate the theoretical issues discussed. *[Article copies available for a fee from The Haworth Document Delivery Service: 1-800-342-9678. E-mail address: <getinfo@haworthpressinc.com> Website: <http://www.HaworthPress.com> © 2001 by The Haworth Press, Inc. All rights reserved.]*

Dr. Isaac Tylim, PsyD, ABPP (Diplomate in Psychoanalysis), is a training analyst of the International Psychoanalytic Association; fellow and faculty member of the Institute for Psychoanalytic Training and Research; faculty member and supervisor of the Institute for Child, Adolescent, and Family Studies; and faculty member and supervisor of the New York University Postdoctoral Program in Psychoanalysis and Psychotherapy. He is also Assistant Professor of Psychiatry, Downstate Medical Center; Adjunct Clinical Assistant Professor of Psychiatry, St. George University Medical School; Coordinator of In-Patient Psychology, Maimonides Medical Center, Brooklyn, NY; Secretary of the International Psychoanalytic Committee on the United Nations; and President Elect, Section I, APA Division 39 (Psychoanalysis). A psychoanalytic film critic, Dr. Tylim publishes regular reviews and essays on contemporary films. He was part of the program committee on the first conference on Film and Psychoanalysis, which was held in Los Angeles in 1995. Dr. Tylim is in private practice in New York City, where he works with individuals, couples, and groups.

Author note: I want to thank Robert Marchesani for editorial comments, and for sharing Marilyn Monroe's quote.

[Haworth co-indexing entry note]: "One Sings, the Other Doesn't: Stage Fright and the Psychoanalytic Theater." Tylim, Isaac. Co-published simultaneously in *The Psychotherapy Patient* (The Haworth Press, Inc.) Vol. 11, No. 3/4, 2001, pp. 11-25; and: *Frightful Stages: From the Primitive to the Therapeutic* (ed: Robert B. Marchesani, and E. Mark Stern) The Haworth Press, Inc., 2001, pp. 11-25. Single or multiple copies of this article are available for a fee from The Haworth Document Delivery Service [1-800-342-9678, 9:00 a.m. - 5:00 p.m. (EST). E-mail address: getinfo@haworthpressinc.com].

KEYWORDS. Psychodynamic, transformation, performance, actors, imposters, exposure, perception, hypochondriasis, audience, spontaneity, resistances, dreams

It had started snowing. But I felt as warm as if I were standing in a bright sun . . . I've always been frightened by an audience–any audience. My stomach pounds, my head gets dizzy and I'm sure my voice has left me. But standing in the snowfall facing these yelling soldiers, I felt for the first time in my life no fear at all. I felt only happy.

–Marilyn Monroe

Stage fright has been defined as a state of morbid anxiety which disturbs the sense of poise (Kaplan, 1995). The affected sense of poise has overt manifestations characterized by severe autonomic responses accompanied by a disorganizing and disorienting effect. During a theatrical performance, the disturbance may last a few minutes or the length of the performance. From a psychodynamic perspective, the actor's loss of the sense of poise may produce a disequilibrium between a need for narcissistic supplies (including recognition and approval from the audience), and the actor's low expectations regarding the nature of the audience's feed-back.

A brief glimpse into the underlying dynamics of this relatively common condition reveals an inability to modulate or regulate affects in front of an audience–that big dark mouth (theater as cavity)–that expects to be fed. Performance anxiety appears as a consequence of the discrepancy between strong oral cravings and limited hope regarding their fulfillment. Kaplan refers to the actor's state of "appetitive arousal" which is stimulated by every performance. According to Gabbard (1983), stage fright is a universal experience of performers and others who stand before an audience. It is also evident whenever one tries something new–for instance, driving a car on the highway for the first time, entering a cocktail party, etc. Repeated experiences may bring a sense of mastery, and anxiety may be dissolved or not be as pronounced.

Actors' stage fright differs significantly from other manifestations of the symptom. Senior professional actors report experiencing stage fright before each show, despite the years of playing the same role. Rituals, obsessive compulsive features, somatizations, and other signifiers of narcissistic regressions are often common back stage, pre-show actions. For instance, Marlene Dietrich used to clean her own dressing room and made sure the stage was properly vacuumed before each performance; well-known actors are notorious for getting drunk in their dressing rooms before going on stage; an actor in psychoanalytic treatment for several years had the entire cast hold hands before curtain call so "the good energy" could be shared.

How does one explain these distressful symptoms in seasoned, well-trained professionals? How is it that repeated exposure to the dreaded object does not contribute much to the transformation of anxiety or to a more adaptive affective regulation? Before going on stage actors may worry about the perception of others. They anticipate and fear that which they hope to evoke in the internal world of the spectator may be absent. In other words, the performer is invested in appearing in a particular way to its audience, e.g., Hamlet as melancholic; the fear is that they might not. The fantasized scenario of failing to do so becomes the source of anxiety which may set up a chain of events which could only be halted by a drastic solution. Under these circumstances, the actor is unable to differentiate fantasy from reality, play from work, pretending from just being in the 'real' world.

Good actors, like good impostors, are masters of imitation. Not unlike impostors, actors perform actions in an aura of pretense. Anxiety about projecting melancholia on stage may betray the actor's fear of not being able to pretend or imitate a melancholic, revealing instead that which must remain hidden or off stage, i.e., the actor's personality, his 'real' being in the world. This 'real' being in the world is often far removed from the character portrayed on stage, and is prone to mobilize unresolved conflicts or tensions between the necessity to deceive in order to act and the inability to do so. In this regard, impostors' tendencies are to be placed in a continuum which ranges from least pathological manifestations, such as those displayed by actors and all those in the creative arts, to the most disturbed patients suffering from narcissistic pathology and/or severe identity disturbance (Gediman & Lieberman, 1996).

Greenacre (1958) considered all impostors as derivations of family romance fantasies. Impostors long to return to childhood omnipotence, that which grown-ups must relinquish. Impostors, like actors, need an audience to confirm the reality of their assumed identity. Yet, actors and impostors belong to two different groups. Actors get anxious, while impostors do not. Impostors have a choice to perform socially or not, while actors must go on stage once they hear the curtain call. Impostoring is close to perversions; performers, on the contrary, do not necessarily function at the level of perverts. In Kaplan's words, performers are "honest men." Performers suffering from stage fright may feel as if they are being tested every time they must go on stage. If they manage to go on with the show, the sense of getting away with incompetence overwhelms them. Gedimann and Lieberman (1996) talk about actors as impostors in reverse or "those who wrongly believe they are impostors." They are fueled by the belief that they are fraudulent, fearing that sooner or later they will be found out. The catastrophic discovery, as far as the performer goes, may lead to public shame and humiliation. Humiliation is the result of the failure of the performer to collude with the audience. Pretense does not work.

Stage fright either benefits or impedes a performance. When functioning as a signal of impending danger, defenses against the interference of "reality" may be mobilized, so the performance may go on smoothly. Stage fright as signal anxiety allows the full immersion of the actor into the "neo" reality of the stage, facilitating the necessary dissociation or depersonalization which accompanies every good performance.

Stage fright may transform itself into severe inhibition. Under these conditions the actor's function becomes compromised. The necessary capacity to dissociate or depersonalize fails. In these cases anxieties pertaining to different levels of psychosexual development often coexist. Exhibitionist aims couple with the need to be recognized by the mirroring eye of the pleased audience; fear of losing control and making a mess on stage manifests anal conflicts and related aggressive themes; too much guilt may inhibit performance since, in order to perform, an attitude of triumph over guilt must prevail.

A manic flight with the inherent denial of childhood limitations allows actors to hold on to the narcissistic omnipotence. But unlike the delusional patient or the psychotic one, the actor has a way of re-entering reality which is dictated by the role, the props, the frame of the text. Rationalizations may be cover-ups for those compromise formations (the symptoms) that help to keep the original conflict out of consciousness. For instance, a talented actor in my practice manages to miss auditions and rehearsals. He finds fault with fellow actors or directors, becoming choosy about roles offered to him. On more than one occasion he has refused to accept promising parts in Broadway shows, claiming that the "character was not well developed." He then proceeds to tell me how comfortable he feels at his restaurant job where the tips are good and the pressure minimal.

What are the differences between inhibitions or phobias and stage fright? Stage fright, unlike inhibitions or phobias, is–as Kaplan puts it–an "induced anxiety state by virtue of the fact that the performer, unlike the neurotic, defies the phobic situation in pursuit of some subsequent advantage." In other words, while the neurotic manages to avoid anxiety through inhibition of behavior, the performer induces it by his wish to perform. The reality of the scheduled performance triggers stage fright. Thus stage fright appears at the threshold where reality must be forgone for the sake of operating in a different reality, that of make believe, the performance.

An attraction to the danger of exposure is often a necessary ingredient of a performance. A counterphobic attitude is the by-product of an optimal, manageable degree of anxiety. Kaplan (1995) stated that the counterphobic dynamic is set up by a possessive and challenging mother who devalues the father and presents him as defective. The child then is forced to overcome his imperfect and ineffectual father with counterphobic measures. The failure to do so, that is in developing counterphobic strategies, leads to a paralyzing stage fright with catastrophic consequences since the performer can't perform.

The ability to move from one conscious state to the other, that is to say from being off stage to being on stage, is too difficult for certain performers whose boundaries are not firmly established. The sense of self is often compromised in these cases in which performers become prey to their fear of losing the grasp they so tenuously held while on stage. Some creative individuals hold on to the organizing reality provided by the "make believe" setting, while failing to function in the reality of everyday life.

During stage fright episodes one may note the prevalence of hypochondriacal features. These are signs of a split between affects and ideation. The body talks in a quasi-symbolic fashion about the distress associated with the exposure. The body becomes a stage where the individual produces the drama of exposure and humiliation. The pregenital aims thus revealed, with their aggressive and libidinal aspects, foster the emergence of annihilation anxiety and fear of dying. (The patient D, discussed below, was afraid of having a heart attack while singing.)

An overall paranoid ambience is created. The body and the mind are both in danger. Hypochondriasis and delusions are both manifestations of paranoid formations. In hypochondriasis the danger is experienced as coming from within; in delusions danger is projected on the external world–the audience–which is expected to devalue or ridicule the performance. And the most terrifying component is that once on the stage, no escape is possible.

From a Kleinian perspective, for the performance to take place, a shift from the paranoid position to the depressive position has to occur. The actor must recreate the character in the depth of his/her internal world. The work of art, whether a painting, a piece of music, an opera, can only be delivered under the guides of reparative mechanisms. Indeed it is through reparation that symbolization occurs. Segal (1991) thinks that the means by which the artist captures and engages the audience is contingent on an attempted resolution of a depressive conflict–reparation. Reparation must include an acknowledgment of aggression and its effect. In this aspect lies the imperfection of a work of art. Actors who strive for perfection cannot resolve the depressive conflict, often getting stuck in the paranoid position under a disguise of stage fright.

The ability to accept imperfections allows the actor to perform the same piece over and over. The re-creation of the production is the beauty of art that gives birth to a new form out of the old, a new Hamlet every few years. Here, in the creation of the new, lie the reparative forces.

The fear of losing control over one's expressive powers is, in my estimation, more pronounced in singers. Singers wear two hats, one as performers, the other as singers. This duality produces both a beneficial and a detrimental effect on the psyche. As performers, improvisation is often possible. Actors, when they forget their lines, make them up based on the context of the production. Improvisation for singers is not that simple. A false note and you are caught. One doesn't have to possess musical skills in order to detect mistakes.

The case of D illustrates Gabbard's assertion (1979) that any conflict in a given performer's stage fright is related to the early childhood experience of that particular performer. During the psychoanalytic process the analyst functions as both the audience and backstage support to the analysand's performance. The analysand lying on the couch experiences the analyst/audience/coach as back there in the dark, watching the show.

THE ANALYSIS OF D

D, a 42-year-old opera singer, entered psychoanalytic treatment over four years ago because he was unable to sing. Married, a father of two young children, he described "an overwhelming anxiety crawling into my body while performing on stage." A graduate of a prestigious music school, D had earned distinguished scholarships and was the recipient of numerous awards. Insightful, with a unique sensitivity to the nuances of his emotional world, D wondered about the psychological nature of his symptoms. He was puzzled by them and wished the analyst could "extract his neurotic inhibitions like a dentist extracts a tooth–fast and without too much pain." He complained of severe throat distress while attempting to sing during a recent rehearsal: "My mouth went dry, I panicked then and ran out of the theater." D was convinced that singing had the potential to irremediably damage his body. This believed threat to his physical integrity fueled experiences of humiliation when he was in front of conductors, colleagues, and critics.

The eloquent and formal presentation of this patient, with the neurotic appreciation of his inhibitions (stage fright), induced in the analyst a fantasy of attending to a classical analytic patient belonging to another place and another time: Vienna, late nineteenth century. Like there and then, the patient agreed to a 4-times-a-week treatment after two consultation sessions. He seemed to welcome the couch as an unquestionable requirement.

D came from an artistic family. Mother was a talented but reclusive writer who, all through her life, refused to publish her work or sell it. She died two years prior to the beginning of the analysis. Prone to severe depressive episodes, Mother was hospitalized for several months when D was two-and-a-half years old. After a trial on medications, she received electric convulsive therapy. The paternal grandmother, a retired singer, took over the running of the house. D described his grandmother as "a warm, dedicated, and supportive soul, always there for me." Father was a music lover who encouraged D to pursue his operatic vocation with a blunt, stern, and hypercritical attitude about his son's strengths and limitations. The oldest of three siblings, D was Mother's favorite, a reliable source of support to her, particularly when Father initiated an affair with a younger woman, abdicating family responsibilities. Mother would cry on D's shoulders, expecting him to take over household chores and the care of the younger siblings. D's parents divorced during his adolescence. D's brother and sister, 2 and 4 years younger than he, established a stronger bond with Father, who, according to D, allowed them "to escape my mother's heavy depressive web."

While talking about his siblings, D had the need to minimize his resentment for their decision to distance themselves from what they perceived as Mother's excessive dependency needs and unbearable clinging. He couldn't comprehend the intensity of the anger his siblings harbored against Mother. D would find himself repeatedly arguing on her behalf or defending her, blaming his father for Mother's "pathetic state." He described Mother as "a mute victim, abandoned by a selfish man for a much younger woman." Eventually D was to assume the responsibility for the care of his dying mother when she contracted a terminal illness.

Early in treatment the patient seemed reluctant to talk or share his thoughts with the analyst. He tended to censor his productions, scanning his mind for the "relevant things you probably expect of me." He often felt foolish and self-conscious, lacking words to express his feelings. The analyst's suggestion to bring up whatever was crossing his mind was often met with a guarded and protective attitude: "I know what you want. You are trying to provoke me so I could make a fool of myself in here." He suspected the analyst was setting him up for some kind of "therapy game" that he couldn't quite figure out. D was convinced that analysis must follow a pre-established order, not unlike a theater production. The analytic setting with its props (couch, the big chair behind, the dimmed lights) conformed to a stage where he was expected to perform in front of an "out of sight" audience–the analyst with his hypercritical ear. D's resistances left no room for spontaneity in his discourse, intellectualizing the process and referring to his acquired knowledge of analytic procedures based on movies and television shows. The analyst pointed out how D felt uncomfortable with the freedom offered by the analysis, adding that "perhaps as a performer you are used to rehearsed scripts . . . without them, you seem lost, afraid of what might come out in the session." With his silence, D was invoking in the transference bath the harsh Father image and the demanding Mother. At times the analyst was accused of attempting to destroy the idealized maternal representation, conspiring with Father "in spoiling my good memories of her."

An early dream illustrates the nature of D's anxiety and resistances. In the dream D sees himself in a public bathroom, trying to urinate. Aware of a presence next to him, he turns around and realizes that someone is watching him. D associated to his uneasiness when having to use a toilet at a recent social function. "When you have to go, you have to go," he remarked. With the analyst's assistance the patient was able to discover the connection between the dream and the analytic situation. The analyst suggested that D was somewhat perplexed about how much control he felt he had to exert during the sessions, despite his knowing that "when you have to go, you have to go." The analyst was like an intrusive presence on the public toilet of the session. It upset D's narcissistic equilibrium "to be watched like that . . . you move and make noises, too much activity in back of me reminds me of being on stage and the crew backstage ambulating while the show is on!"

D's curiosity about what was going on in back of the couch preoccupied him. He became almost obsessed with the inner work of the analysis and the vicissitudes of the analytic process. He wanted to peep into the analyst's privacy in order to grasp "what analysis was really about." "Tell me about your training?" he would ask. "How do you professionals know when you are ready to call yourselves analysts?" He ruminated on the problems of confidentiality, worrying about the analyst sharing information with others, or about the press finding out he was in treatment. Exhibitionistic urges alternated with voyeuristic ones. The analyst was watching the analysand watching the analyst, or the analysand was watching the analyst watching the analysand; performer and audience taking turns in a narcissistic reflection of the analytic theater.

The hot days of June offered D an opportunity to expand on the effects changes in the weather had on him. He was reading about the depletion of ozone and its relevance to the hot New York summers.

D: I am praying for rain, I can't stand this heat. . . . It's been so dry. A state of emergency may be declared if it doesn't rain soon. It is hard to sing when it gets too hot. Your mouth dries up.

A: Like the weather now, you too are going through a dry spell. Your mouth gets dry and you can't 'sing' either on stage or on the couch. If you don't 'sing,' a state of emergency may be declared in your analysis.

D began then to explore the meaning of "dry" and "wet." Well into the fall, the rains arrived. Soaked, wearing boots and holding a drooling umbrella, patient entered my wall-to-wall carpeted office and reclined on the couch without giving me time to stop his wet advances. He became apologetic when I asked him to remove his boots and jacket. He remained mute for the rest of the hour. The analyst's intervention was rather minimal: "You are trying to tell me that the dry period is over."

D: I guess so, now I have no more excuses.

A shift took place in the analysis. Lateness, cancellations, missing appointments followed. Not without opposition, D accepted my invitation to analyze the "wet incident." He felt reprimanded by the statement about the dry period.

D: I know it's irrational, but you made me feel like a little boy. I felt so embarrassed. I don't understand why. I guess I was messing up your couch and carpet. I am usually good about these things, I mean order and neatness. The way you looked at me when I stood up to remove my boots and jacket. . . .

A: You finally were able to 'sing' in my presence, and you worried about spoiling the office and me with what may come out. And then my look of disapproval frightened you, as if this time you were urinating in front of me.

On one occasion D brought in a piece of music paper. Over musical notes he wrote a few words reminding himself of something he was determined to share with the analyst: "A recollection I had on my way home after the last session . . . I remembered getting into a fight with a boy who lived next door. Afraid of the much bigger boy, I ran as fast as I could, scared, my heart pounding, hoping to find safe refuge at home. Instead, I realized that my mother had witnessed the scene through the window of her bedroom. 'You are a coward D,' she jumped on me, turning her back and leaving me hanging." The analyst was becoming a rendition of mother/voyeur, ready to jump on him as Mother did. The threat to the integrity of his body was linked to D's fear of damaging his body while singing. The mysteries of the analytic work were translated into primal scene material with D's sense of exclusion from the domain that belongs to "adults." He expanded on how just recently he had installed a new lock on his bedroom door. His wife insisted on keeping their intruder son out of their privacy. D wanted to understand why he felt so guilty about defining boundaries.

D: It doesn't seem to bother you when my session is over. You simply ask me to leave. With my mother I never knew what role to play. She really teased me. At times I was treated like a special child, a friend or confidant. Then, out of the blue she would turn against me. I could never understand why. It is was very confusing to me.

A: Yes, it must have been very confusing not knowing whether you were your mother's child or your mother's big man.

The meaning of D's writing over musical notes eluded the analyst at that time. Was the patient referring to a symbolic equivalence between singing and telling/talking in sessions? Was he expressing the wish to go back on stage and display his phallic power by singing? "How do you know when you are ready to be an analyst?" D asked again.

A: Do you mean how one knows when one is ready to be a man and feel entitled to have what father had?

D: Yes, that is, you must get me there, I have to grow up. Why is this taking so long? Why am I still afraid?

The theme of looking and being looked at was further elaborated. D brought up revealing associations in this respect. He remembered standing still in front of Mother when she would write for hours during weekends. Mother often used D as the subject of her short stories and novels. D mentioned that her last book was named *The Unfinished Story.* The analyst suggested that perhaps there was 'unfinished' business between D and Mother like there must be 'unfinished' issues between him and his analyst who had just announced his upcoming vacation. D was his analyst's and mother's subject. He was lying there on the couch, still like a well-behaved child. The analyst was about to leave him, interrupting the work in the middle of something important, not unlike Mother with her unfinished story.

During the analyst's vacation the patient visited his father. He reported being uncomfortable with Father who "was making out openly with his young wife in front of my children." D wanted to call attention to this behavior, but hesitated to do so. A cousin had asked him to sing a Christmas song. First he refused, but then thought that "my analyst might want me to." To his surprise he didn't panic and was able to breathe appropriately. "People applauded, I blushed but felt good about my accomplishment. My father, the buster, you know what he said? Your shirt does not go with your trousers! Can you believe it. I take this big step after all this time and he takes it away from me."

A: You wanted to prove that you were not a coward, and your father reminds you that you have a little penis, that the women belong to him, and that you have nothing to sing about.

The interpretation seemed to have facilitated the incursion into D's sexuality, exploring his masturbatory fantasies. Elaborated rituals around baths and showers were the source of D's sexual excitement. He would be turned on by women getting wet during a rain storm, picturing himself making love to a half dressed woman whose clothes were soaked. Castration anxieties were analyzed in the context of D's fetishistic practices. The contamination of genitality by pre-genital urges became more apparent while the earlier "dry-wet" dichotomy was revisited in light of the new material.

To sing was D's attempt to prove he was a grown-up man, possessor of a penis capable of matching his father's. The danger of showing off his penis led to stage fright and subsequent inhibition of his capacity to perform. At this point in the analysis, D started to bring up material he once thought was irrelevant to the analysis. He revealed that for years he has been collecting hats, "all kinds, big hats." When Father sees him wearing a hat, he often teases him, at times tossing the hat into the air. D described his various moods while wearing hats.

D: I feel I am able to assume a persona, like when on the stage. . . . When I sing, the one that sings is a persona, a mask, not the real me. The real me is inside, mute like my mother when she was depressed. She couldn't talk. She used to stare at me, with those bovine eyes.

A: One part of you sings; the other doesn't, being too wrapped up with your mother's sadness.

At this point tears began to flow over his cheeks. The analyst remained silent while D sobbed. Before leaving the session the patient remarked with a smile: "I am all wet again."

The "unfinished story" introduced the image of a mother who seldom completed household chores or tasks. As a child, D remembered setting up the table, doing the dishes, cleaning up after Mother. He conveyed the image of a depressed woman who gravitated to her studio or her bedroom, going days at the time without talking.

D: There were days that she wouldn't come down. I kept my siblings busy while she was alone in her room. I felt sorry for her. She seemed so sad. My father ignored her altogether. But I must admit liking being needed, it made me feel important.

A: You became the man of the house, and perhaps you thought you could do a better job than your father.

D: The truth is that I was doing a better job . . . which also left me with a feeling that I was getting away with something. . . .

Towards the beginning of the third year of his treatment, he brought up a childhood incident which had haunted him for years. His mother decided to adopt her eight-year-old nephew whose mother had died suddenly. D, five years old at the time, recalled how rejected he felt, beginning to entertain fantasies of revenge. This recollection appeared to be a screen memory for D's humiliation and betrayal following the birth of his brother. For the first time the patient understood that his mother's depression around the time his brother was born must have been diagnosed as a post-partum depression. D had lost his mother twice: to her depression, and to his brother. The adopted cousin shared a room with D and his siblings for many years. One night D caught him stealing money from his brother. Running to his mother he told her what he saw. Mother decided then to place the nephew in a home for adolescent boys. D felt guilty for having been an informer, telling on an orphan, 'singing' the truth. Once again, D experienced the analytic sessions as a place where he was forced to 'sing,' to tell on others, to be an informer. D couldn't hide from the analyst's scrutiny as he couldn't hide from the audience while on stage. The murderous rage at his little brother seems to have been displaced towards his cousin. Unearthing D's depressed aggression appeared to disorganize him. Lacking words to express himself, D felt filled with bodily sensations he couldn't control, as if his mother were crawling inside his body preventing him from singing.

PROCESS NOTES FROM TWO CONSECUTIVE SESSIONS

D: I am worried about my son. We just received a letter from the Dean. He wants to meet with my wife and me. I keep a long list of good and bad things my son does, an inventory. He is so needy, my boy. Despite spending a lot of time doing things together, nothing seems to be enough for him . . . and yet I feel guilty, responsible for his problems at school. I don't know what I can do differently . . . (long pause). Last night I had this dream: my daughter was sitting on the toilet wearing a party dress. She was actually inside the toilet. She didn't appear to be upset. I told her not to touch anything. That's all I remember. . . . We went to a party on Sunday. My daughter was wearing a beautiful party dress. She looked like a little adult and she talked like one. In many ways she is more self-sufficient and outgoing than my son. Actually I think the dream is about him. My daughter socializes, interacts with others, moves around; my son clings more to me. He sat next to me the whole evening. I love him very much, but at times it is exasperating. He is a big boy, almost an adolescent . . . and still he wants to hold my hand. . . .

A: You are telling me you are a big boy now. You are back on stage, singing. You wish to let go of my hand and do things on your own. Perhaps you feel there is something unclean about the analysis, this toilet where you may be touched by a man.

D: It is true. I must confess that in here I feel both like a man and like a boy. You are right about that. A man should be independent, take the bull by the horns. I am pushing my son to go out, to travel around the city with public transportation. . . . I want to do my own thing, away from you. Yesterday I was singing 'big' music. It felt great. My mouth was open, filled with notes. Thanks to the analysis I am now capable of understanding the differences between emotional problems that interfere with my performances and the technical pieces. At times, while singing, curses, bad words are crossing my mind. Also this thought occurs to me: what if I lose my breathing? What if I breathe the wrong away and cause damage to my body? It does happen to singers you know? Yet recently beautiful women began to appear while I daydream backstage. I wonder why.

A: Some of those emotional problems may interfere with your performance here. You want space from me, to be on your own, and you have trouble expressing your anger at needing me. It must be hard to sing with curses in your mind.

D: Anger always gets in my way. . . . At times I am so tough with my son.

He is a good artist. You know, his drawings are about people in armor . . . just like my drawings used to be. As a child I used to write violent stories. My father once discovered them and he punished me for them. I couldn't show them to my mother either. She would've been infuriated. She was the writer, not me. I felt corralled. No place to go with my anger. I had to sing in my room when nobody was around, and also I had to hide my writing. . . . Before going away to school I destroyed all my writing. You probably think I didn't want to compete with my mother. . . . I think it was more out of rage and how oppressive she was. . . . Have you kept the poems I brought to you? Have you stored them in my file? Where do you keep your files? I may want them back someday.

A: You want me to know that they are your poems. Like your singing is your singing. You value them now.

D: I do, I am in that mode as of late. What's mine is precious. I am giving myself permission to enjoy my fantasies. . . .

THE FOLLOWING SESSION

D: The days are longer. I love the summer, particularly the evenings. The music of nature, the colors of the city. I may be singing in Philadelphia, then upstate. I am wondering whether it will be a large auditorium. I guess it is OK to feel some degree of anxiety about it. You told me so . . . listen to this dream: I am rehearsing. The opera score is in front of me. The words are in Latin. Over the score someone drew clouds. I find it hard to read. The conductor seems impatient . . . I need help with Latin. Why Latin?

A: What about Latin?

D: Latin is like a sacred language used for special occasions. The priest knows it, not the congregation. I felt pressured by the conductor . . . as if he wanted me to move on, to go for it, but I was somewhat reluctant. I hesitated. Reminds me of yesterday. I got this phone call. A guy was asking me to donate blood. He was so insistent. I was getting annoyed. People want to absorb you. He wouldn't let go.

A: You want to sing but can't read the music. The clouds are an obstruction, hiding the sun, the music. . . . To perform is like giving out your blood, giving away something precious to you. Like your poems. Perhaps you are not sure whether I would return them to you?

D: No, it isn't just that. I have to conform when I sing. I resent this to an extent. I like to be different from those people that conform. I must be in the wrong profession. Look at my brother or sister. They always did what they wanted to do. I am still dependent in so many ways, on my teachers, my analysis, air-supply. . . . Intelligence? I don't need intelligence in order to sing. I have witnessed individuals whose intellects were inferior to mine yet became great singers. . . . I feel as if someone has given me a splendid golden watch in a thousand pieces, and my task was to put these pieces together without knowing much about watchmaking. . . . Time keeps its bit whether or not the clock is ever assembled. . . . And ironically I am singing again. . . . This is so confusing.

A: Time goes on and you feel that the analysis hasn't put all the pieces together. You are singing and you may have to terminate the analysis with a valuable golden watch still not completely assembled. A kind of unfinished novel.

D: (eyes are watering, long pause) I remember my mother trying to teach me Madame Butterfly . . . I must have been 10 or 11 years old. Listening to the record over and over. My father must've been out of the house, who knows. She needed me.

A: And you needed him to help you deal with your mother's pain.

D: She must've been suicidal then. Three kids and a philandering husband.

A: Madame Butterfly and her only, special child.

D: I always thought that Madame Butterfly was a very sick woman.

D has recently begun to audition for several national and international companies. No contracts yet, but he feels more comfortable on stage, confident that he'll soon be touring again. He reported a dream where he was taking a master class with an old teacher he knew very well. The class was to be the last one before opening night. He was trying to finish learning a difficult aria, anxious that he was running out of time. D reported having seen the play "Master Class" which he enjoyed tremendously. When the analyst inquired about what he so much enjoyed about the play, he described the title scene where a bright student rebels against the demanding and condescending teacher (Maria Callas), and storms out of the room.

D: (eyes are getting teary) New York in the summer . . . the evenings are golden . . . I feel I am entering the sunset of my career. Beautiful like a sunset, but a sunset nonetheless. The kids are out of school. It makes me sad. Another year.

A: Perhaps it is the sunset of the analysis that is making you sad.

D: Could you hand the tissues to me . . . I don't have a handkerchief in my pocket. You see how dependent on you I still am. I need your tissues. Outside of here I feel like a thief. I steal your ideas or comments and use them to understand others. I borrow things from you like in Cyrano. You are Cyrano . . . I rely on your words. (long pause)

The dream presents some elements of the terminal phase of the analysis (about to finish the aria). D wonders how he will part from the analysis. The analyst's omnipotence is being challenged (the student confronts Maria Callas). On one occasion the patient wore dark glasses while entering into the consultation room. One may understand this acting out as a form of detachment or need to distance himself from the analyst. D seemed invested in protecting himself against the possibility of a premature termination, or rather interruption, of his analysis.

Will D's analysis become like Mother's unfinished story? Has the patient fulfilled his wish of the analyst extracting his symptom fast and without pain? Or is the patient engaged in a form of repetition of his connection to Mother and her unfinished story? Is this resorting to action a means of by-passing the painful working through and the concomitant mourning that may be necessary to complete "the unfinished story/analysis"? Countertransferentially, the analyst may have to mourn the loss of such a good patient who reminds him of a nineteenth century Viennese one. The mourning in the analyst finds expression in his renewed interest in listening to operas. Like Mother who couldn't let go of either her son or her novels, the analyst may have trouble letting go of the patient. Further exploration of the vicissitudes of transference and countertransference phenomena may still be awaiting in the near future. However, one should not ignore the effect that an out-of-town singing contract may have on the fate of this analysis. In this regard, the analyst's fantasies of being irreplaceable have to be closely monitored.

REFERENCES

Greenacre, P. (1958). The relation of the impostor to the artist. Psychoanalytic Study of the Child 13: 2-36.

Gediman, H.K. & Lieberman, J.S. (1996). The Many Faces of Deceit. Northvale, N.J.: Jason Aronson Inc.

Gabbard, G.O. (1979). Stage fright. International Journal of Psychoanalysis, 60: 383-392.

Gabbard, G.O. (1983). Further contributions to the understanding of stage fright: Narcissistic Issues. Journal of the American Psychoanalytic Association, 31: 423-441.

Kaplan, D. (1995). Stage fright. In Clinical and Social Realities, ed. L. Kaplan. Northvale, NJ: Jason Aronson Inc.

Segal, H. (1991). Dream, Phantasy, and Art. London: Tavistock/Routledge.

The Awesome and the Awestruck: Bessie Smith and Carl Van Vechten

E. Mark Stern

SUMMARY. In this essay, an attempt is made to describe the heartland of the invidiously awestruck. Historical accounts blend in with ersatz translations of key events without abandoning the qualitative interaction between the two principal characters, Carl Van Vechten, the pursuer, and Bessie Smith, the distancer. Against these figures, brief suggestions are made for a psychotherapy of allowing awe to be what it is, even if it be unbearable, while moving into a greater realization of one's own potentials. *[Article copies available for a fee from The Haworth Document Delivery Service: 1-800-342-9678. E-mail address: <getinfo@haworthpressinc. com> Website: <http://www.HaworthPress.com> © 2001 by The Haworth Press, Inc. All rights reserved.]*

KEYWORDS. Harlem Renaissance, race relations, alienating boundaries, visual arts, music

The opera was from the start an education less musical than sentimental. We were the puppets! Why else had we paid . . . to hear Violetta suffer? . . . Flagstad's Brunnhilde stood out larger than life. . . . Next to

E. Mark Stern, EdD, ABPP (Diplomate in Clinical Psychology), is a Fellow of the American Psychological Association, the American Psychological Society, and the Academy of Clinical Psychology. He is Emeritus Professor, Graduate School of Arts and Sciences at Iona College in New Rochelle, New York. Dr. Stern is in private practice of psychotherapy in New York City and Clinton Corners in Dutchess County, NY.

[Haworth co-indexing entry note]: "The Awesome and the Awestruck: Bessie Smith and Carl Van Vechten." Stern, E. Mark. Co-published simultaneously in *The Psychotherapy Patient* (The Haworth Press, Inc.) Vol. 11, No. 3/4, 2001, pp. 27-35; and: *Frightful Stages: From the Primitive to the Therapeutic* (ed: Robert B. Marchesani, and E. Mark Stern) The Haworth Press, Inc., 2001, pp. 27-35. Single or multiple copies of this article are available for a fee from The Haworth Document Delivery Service [1-800-342-9678, 9:00 a.m. - 5:00 p.m. (EST). E-mail address: getinfo@haworthpressinc.com].

the powers of such a woman, all male activity–Siegfried's dragon slay-
ing, Einstein's theorizing, the arcana of password and sweat ledge-
seemed tame and puerile.

–James Merrill

Love is giving something you haven't got to someone who doesn't
exist.

–Jacques Lacan

O mother of the hills, forgive our towers;
O mother of the clouds, forgive our dreams.

–Edwin Ellis

The awestruck elude facile diagnosis. The most admiring of them venerate
the idyllic. Others, less given to inner resources, are drawn to inaccessible
human icons. These are inebriated with an awe that subjects them to pro-
longed periods of excitement and frustration. Some stalk while others invade
boundaries. All fail to differentiate between the golden calf and the golden
boy.

Awe that is invidiously jealous annuls Saint Paul's admonition that "Love
envieth not." In such covetousness, the spirit of Dionysian excess prevails
for ill fortune. The grasping grip of such awe heightens the passions even as
its adherents push to consume their beloved.

Semi-fact tells the story of two erstwhile public figures:

- Carl Van Vechten: man of letters and unique talents; awe-stricken admirer.
- Bessie Smith: fiery chanteuse; alone in the galaxy; empress of the
  blues; idolized.

These two ingenious figures linger in the echoes of bygone gossip. So I
too take bold strokes of liberty with the literal accuracy of events. This is
about the phenomenon of idolizing awe.

Carl Van Vechten was born on June 17, 1880, in Cedar Rapids, Iowa,
thirteen years after his next oldest sibling. By the time of Carl's birth, his
parents, active radicals engrossed in the struggle for equality and fairness for
women and Afro-Americans, were well into their forties. Foretelling some of
his own interest, Carl's father was a co-founder of the first Black school in
Mississippi.

From childhood on Carl was embarrassed by his awkward appearance. He was gawky, a lad six feet tall by the time he was thirteen, and warped through his growing sensitive years by protruding front teeth. Self detesting, Carl tortured himself even more by resorting to constructing crude fillers made up of thick rubber bands in countless failed attempts at homebred orthodontia. Carl, like generations of the self-loathing, wanted to be what he was not.

Carl attended the University of Chicago, where he earned a Bachelor's degree in the visual arts and music. The university afforded him an excellent opportunity to become familiar with Chicago's emerging cultural life. Soon after graduating, he landed a reporter's job at the *American*. Despite his quick wit and talent with words, the work of a journalist soon became mundane. Carl, a mutineer at heart, was hell-bent on subverting what he experienced as the imprint of propriety. Assigned to cover a horse show, Carl facetiously described the gauche frivolities of the frenzied audience. Finding himself thinking more about the social jungle than insignificant events, Carl was promptly dismissed from the paper. The young man moved on to New York City where a better life hopefully awaited him. Drawing on his cosmopolitan talents, Carl scored a post as music and arts critic for Theodore Dreiser's *Broadway Magazine*. In a matter of months he was asked to relocate abroad as the publication's foreign correspondent. While in Europe, he married an old school chum. The union was short lived. But while still together, the couple made numerous social connections with such luminaries as Gertrude Stein and the art and literary expatriate scene. A few years later, now divorced, and once again in New York, Carl was on his way to making his mark as an astute music critic.

Although openly homosexual, Carl remarried. The new Mrs. Van Vechten was the spirited Russian actress Fania Marinoff. Their close bond survived bottles of chilled white wines and perilous escapades for well over 50 years.

Carl's relentless restlessness was cut, in part, to the pattern of his family's social consciousness. He seemed endlessly and equally to be in search of the eminently prominent and the socially besieged. Carl was the intrepid besieger. This quixotic temperament blended well with his mischievous and gregarious propensities. Carl learned the exquisite skills of the more successful of the charming gadabouts. Musician and novelist Paul Bowles (1972, p. 340) recalls one of his rare visits to New York. On that occasion, he happened to meet Carl on a random street. He wanted to know if there was anyone in the whole of the city Paul wanted to meet. "Meet?" answered a bewildered Bowles. Carl's response was instant and boundlessly excited: "I mean is there anyone you don't know that you'd like to know?" Out of a hat, Bowles mentioned James Purdy, a recently celebrated short-story writer. "Come (to my apartment) Wednesday evening at seven." As expected, there was an obedient Purdy, come to call on command. Carl, who had by now perfected the role of observer, snapped countless pictures of the strangers, but in the style of the two having long known each other. Carl became a novelist much in the way he had perfected his brand of photography. There was a trans-migration of intimacy in both of these expressive forms–Carl, the adoring admirer, with a growing reputation for making ample use of allies and enemies in his artistic endeavors.

Much was happening to bring high hopes. The great Harlem Renaissance was now in its stunning emergence. This was the quintessential time of awakening for many Black artists, writers, and activists. The Renaissance, in all its luster, was hoping to move a people beyond their alienating boundaries. Artists, musicians, and writers alike gathered under the banner of this mobilizing Renaissance. The Renaissance originally grew out of a continuing series of heated exchanges and brotherly handclasps. It marked the rise of the "new Negro" at a time of transplantation from downtown slum communities up to a new homeland in Harlem.

Inspired by the principles of his own family, Carl was easily intoxicated by the emergence of this new Black culture: its paintings, woodcarvings, works in stone and especially its music. Jazz, known more popularly at the time as the "blues," was particularly enchanting to him. He, the archetypal outsider, had found a place of wonder and welcome.

The movement thrived and Carl was soon celebrated as its principal White fellow traveler. Informally, he was to be known as Carlo as he traveled through his new scene. It was not long until he blossomed as one of the innovative novelists, essayists, and photographers of the new Black experience. Walter White, founder of the National Association for the Advancement of Colored People, thought so highly of Van Vechten that he named his first son after him. He won out over his critics, even as his talents were hailed by such famed Black poets as James Weldon Johnson and Langston Hughes. In fact, Langston Hughes lived with the Van Vechtens while composing the poetry for the second edition of Carl's celebrated novel *Nigger Heaven.* As a controversial novel, *Nigger Heaven* had its few detractors in the Black community, though most felt that it was an exceptionally fine depiction of life in the Harlem of the 1920s. This Renaissance ennobled the visions and aesthetics of a Black literati as well as those who were sympathetic to its essence and aesthetic. The movement might have lasted well into the mid-century, but for the end of its utopian vision during the great 1929 Depression.

Somewhere in the thick of the Renaissance, Carl caught sight of blues singer Bessie Smith. Was it the ethic of pity, which was about to take its toll? Bessie was born dirt poor and raised in the shabby corridors of a southern ghetto. Like many kids of the era, she eked out pennies in street performances and in shaky dives. In 1912 she was discovered by the legendary Ma Rainey. She appeared with Ma's company in Chattanooga, Tennessee, where just forty years earlier General Ulysses Grant and his troops marshaled their forces against this struggling Confederate stronghold. Bessie never lost the wounds of growing up Black and poor in the Deep South. Her vulnerability may have been responsible for brandishing her furies. Bessie distrusted Whites. Avenging many accumulated hurts in the years of her successes, she made it policy to hire only the darkest-skinned performers who qualified for a place in her travelling troupe.

For Bessie, the Harlem Renaissance was cloaked in sham. Like other mirages, it was like driving down a long road and getting back to where you started. Besides distrusting those Whites who were a never-ending presence, Bessie most feared the sophisticated Blacks. Bessie avoided New York, deciding instead to make her home in Philadelphia. In Philadelphia one knew where the great racial divide began. Bessie liked to know where she stood.

For Bessie, having to deal with White admirers was a bad scene. Even though she knew that many Whites were drawn to the indigenous rhymes and rhythms of the underclass Blacks, this did not make them any more acceptable to her.

It's hard to date when Bessie became popularly known as "The Empress of the Blues." There was good and there was bad to any coronation. The Empress's talents frequently shrieked into blind rampages. Blistering furies echoed their way into countless wild sexual liaisons with an unloving assortment of titillating male and female gigolos. A series of aborted marriages added to her mind-set of grisly trophies. Tragic as her life had been, Bessie and her brand of the blues took the pop music world of the 1920s by storm.

Carl Van Vechten was among Bessie's awestruck heralds. He saw in the music that she rendered a complement to his own personification of the eternal outsider. He saw beyond her lavish exterior. But what he saw left him mournfully thirsty. He could sense that her childhood hurts were eternal obstacles to any sort of friendship. He who had made friends with the grandest of the Black literati was nevertheless dazzled by the rejecting tone of Bessie's occult never-to-be-possessed presence. Her golden gravel intonations could never abide the persistence of a Prometheus. The more rejected, the more plagued into Byronic submission. Carl was driven to know Bessie. This is how it happened.

Carl's inaugural article for *Vanity Fair* communicates his awe in first encountering Bessie:

> Walking slowly to the footlights . . . she began her strange, rhythmic rites in a voice full of shouting and moaning and praying and suffering, a wild rough Ethiopian voice, harsh and volcanic, but seductive and sensuous too, released between rouged lips and the whitest teeth, the singer, swaying lightly to the beat, as is the Negro custom.
>
> Now inspired by the expressive words, partly by the strain of the accompaniment, partly by the powerfully magnetic personality of this

elemental composed woman with her pleasant African voice, quivering with passion and pain.

In time Bessie would be invited by Carl to one of his grand soirees. A drunken and sometimes opportunistic partying held sway at Carl and Fania's lush New York apartment. In some slight way it might have communicated the flavor of Gertrude Stein's Parisian salon which Carl referred to as a vial of "poisonous darkening drunk (fused with) all the joy in weak success" (Van Vetchen, 1914).

Bessie knew it was in her best interest to resist most social invitations involving the Renaissance. Bessie was understandably distrustful of the crowd that appeared at such gatherings. She had small sympathy for intellectuals, be they Black or White. Bessie reached for her people, with whom she could cope. She was not about to chance anything that would compromise her persona. She preferred audiences that offered her a devoted spiritual linkage. Carl was not one to grasp the idea of boundary. He was susceptible only to the approval of his friends. For Carl, building his community, at any cost, was an evangelic preoccupation. There was no relenting. Bessie knew that the summons was out there. Her managers were convinced that being seen at a Van Vetchen event was in Bessie's best interest. She might at least put in an appearance for the press. And it was true that her musical delivery truly appealed to the new Renaissance.

Carl adored his raven goddess from a world of differences that tantalized and intoxicated his pursuit. Perhaps it was his homosexuality that accounted for his romanticized view of an unavailable woman or perhaps his own history as an anxious voyeur prodded him to move in as close as he could. Carl saw himself as disfigured. Moreover, this impatient onlooker had, more than likely, learned much from the forbidden scenes that attracted him in childhood. In trying to delineate Carl's view of the world, it is important to note that his personal sense of who he was ranged from segments of grandiosity to periods of self-repulsion. I am left to conclude that the people who awed him the most were those who appeared not to have wanted him. In the same sense he was known to fend off those who most cared for him. Some might see Carl's non-sexual, but equally strong desire for the palatine magnificence that Bessie embodied, as way of identifying with the antagonist. Carl was bewitched by attractions, which far outweighed libidinal drive. Bessie's presence, imaginal and mystical as it was, peaked the temptation of the moment. As for Bessie, we know that she shied away from Carl for reasons of her own. She was not about to play gladiator at his festivals. More than likely, Bessie was both awed and disturbed at being cast as an object of worship.

Carl's interest in Bessie left him immobilized. But his ultimate attempts at winning her graces were to become a victory in defeat. Bessie's voice, anointed with a Delilah-like maternal seductiveness, enchanted. Nevertheless, the Philistine Delilah of the Hebrew Bible was to be known as the exceptional woman who was capable of luring the Israelite Samson into losing his exhaustless strength. And in the spirit of Delilah, Bessie was to act out of a sense of impending disaster.

Bessie did show up at the Van Vechten apartment. It was as unexpected as it was surprising. Almost at once, the temperature tightened. It might be termed a tentative fiber of death. More annihilation than disagreeableness. The presence of an unknown sense of the familiar.

Bessie's repeated refills of whisky became obvious. Had she scratched a mosquito bite, it too would have been obvious. No unveiled suspense, but the slow release of flame. The unholy bargain dawned. It was about to be consummated. Bessie began. Blues rolled a wide berth. Fuddled gesticulations, but every phrase a medicament. No medicine for the songster. Her words cried out from anguish: *Dyin' by the Hour*; *Downhearted Blues*; *Saint Louis Woman.* Soon the passion descended into splutters. Diminutive applause. Bessie persevered. Carl, awestruck puer, feasted on endless lamentations. Gin wandered along, peaceful then wrathful. Strains of song freed of all restriction. In the end, Eden turned to fire; transformed into the inferno: *Lost Your Head Blues.* Nothing to transcend. Everything in jeopardy: *Gin House Blues.* In the near end, Bessie's dervish-like balancing act. By now an attentive crowd swooning and dancing in the smallest of movements. But heedless. Bessie was in catastrophe.

Fania knew the fever. She was deeply concerned. This was no mere performance. The capella sistina had moved into an awful ubiquity. Fania moved in ever so closer. She reached out to Bessie. It was a tender signal. The evening must close. You hug a child; you whisper how wonderful she is. Bessie had no way of decoding the message. Love was no ultimate; not even a tiny piece of gratitude, Bessie raged. Fania was thrown to the ground. Carl, aghast as he was, did nothing. He could not transfuse what had happened. Carl procrastinated just long enough. He was prisoner to Bessie's illusions. Fania, bruised and in shock, resumed her own posture without her husband's help or seeming sympathy. He, never abandoning his attraction and craving, knew that it was best to lure his dark visitor out to and into the hallway, and lovingly accompany her to a descending elevator (Douglas, 1995).

Bessie was right to convince herself that she was the one who had been violated; treated no better than an organ grinder's monkey. It was she who had tugged at the lowest branch to find ballast.

Carl could not find it in himself to realize that there had been a violation. His facial cast was grounded, not so much by regret, but by caution. He asked himself if he'd done something he should now be sorry for. Were there sado-masochistic indications that might help shed some light? My hunch is that whatever pain/pleasure complementarity led to Bessie's outburst was not accidental. Rather, both parties played into a consensual tragic/comedic drama. The episode, which appeared to be limitless, had its fine-tuned perimeters. Indeed, what occurred that night appeared to be a social construction in which the romance of aptitudes and cultures volitionally collided. The uproarious tensions had become expressions of how one man and one woman engaged themselves in a creative enterprise of intimacy in which the desexualization of attraction became climactic. True that both Bessie and Van Vechten were long overdue on overcoming feelings of personal insignificance. The impression that Carl and his guests had overstepped Bessie's boundaries and demeaned her dignity might be acknowledged, but only within a political frame of reference. Bessie's reputation for tempestuousness was inherent to her voice. Her artistic appeal could also be tender and affectionate. But the tacit "agreement" of this particular rendezvous was that awe would win out and overlap with the power of the interaction between audience and heroine.

In her role as the object of one man's awe, Bessie slyly enveloped those others who craved as well for their lost innocence. Bessie could indeed identify with Deliah, and in detail and characteristic could as Delilah be the mother of commanding rapture. As with all gods in easy reign, the danger rested with her becoming target for those whose unquenchable desire was to consume her.

Bessie, of course, was much more than her immediacy to those who would personify her as a goddess. The passion of soul makes dynamic the tension of meshing together those for whom the songs are made. Elia Kazan (1988, p. 145) saw this lacework of relationship enfold Bessie into an impassioned spokesperson. Bessie Smith, according to Kazan, "made a league of all the down-and-outers . . . (She) sang for them all and for her race as well." Given her strange mystery of cataclysmic dynamic allure, Bessie's voice erupted into mournful cantorial invocations. This level of awe transformed severe privation into deep prayerful confrontation. *Nobody Knows When You're Down and Out* (1929), the leitmotif of the Great Depression, signaled the abysmal descent of a generation's wild hopes. As the economy disintegrated, so too did the rallying of the Harlem Renaissance vanish and so too did Bessie Smith's career come crashing down. Her tragic end came in an automobile collision in 1937. It happened on the main road to Memphis, just south of her hometown, Clarksdale, Mississippi. Her life might have been saved were it not that the White ambulance driver refused to take her to the nearest hospital. Instead, Bessie's last vestiges of blood flowed with her to her death on the long long journey to the Black infirmary too many miles away to have saved her.

The Bessie/Carl collusion raises issues for psychotherapy. Awe idealizes what it assumes the other person to be. Clients are often in awe of their therapists; and when they are not, they may regard the therapist as the channeling force to the one who is awed. Awe must be treasured even as it keeps the person who experiences it as ambiguous. Awe points one in a direction of "this I must have, though I know that once I find it that explosion may substitute for responsiveness." All are targets as unobtainable heroes. All are hunters of unattainable goals. Recall Caesar who stumbled in pain on his way to die at the feet of the exquisite image of Pompeii.

Adoring the gods violates them. But to never adore; to never love a Bessie; to never contend with a Carl leaves little consolation. Awe is to be endured, even though it can never lead to actual possessiveness. Psychotherapy is beginning to know that the only tenderness rests in distance, but that in distance's absence upheaval is probable.

Carl Van Vechten learned to see and not presume on any but Bessie Smith to claim to discontinuity. There is a piece not told in this essay. Bessie came round to see and be seen by Carl in still another light. She would twinkle like a distant galaxy. And this was good. One day, Bessie agreed that she'd sit for a series of photographic portraits which have become part of a collection of Carl Van Vetchen's works at the United States Library of Congress.

REFERENCES

Bowles, P. (1972) *Without stopping: An autobiography.* New York: The ECCO Press.

Douglas, A. (1995) *Terrible honesty: Mongrel Manhattan in the 1920's.* New York: Noonday.

Hillman, J. (1978) *Myth of analysis: Three essays in archetypal psychology.* New York: Harper & Row.

Hillman, J. (1979) Senex and puer: an aspect of the historical and psychological present in *Puer papers* (edited by Hillman, J. et al.) Irving, TX: Spring Publications (p. 3).

Kazan, E. (1988) *A life.* New York: Alfred A Knopf.

Nugent, C. (1989) *Masks of Satan: The demonic in history.* Westminster MD: Christian Classic.

Van Vechten, C. (1914) How to read Gertrude Stein. *The Trend.* V 01. 7, No. 5 Pp. 553-557.

Van Vechten, C. (1925/1998) *American Decades*–CD Rom. New York: Gale Research.

Burnt Offerings to Prometheus: The Consultation Meetings Between Thomas Merton and Gregory Zilboorg

Alexander Smith

SUMMARY. The unconscious need to idealize another is vividly portrayed in the historical meeting between the famous Catholic writer, Thomas Merton, and Gregory Zilboorg, an important historical figure in American psychiatry. The meetings in 1956 grew out of Merton's personal crisis with his monastic vocation and Zilboorg's presumption to resolve it. In the context of consultation with religious communities, the meetings richly illustrate the ease with which we can distort the greatness of another, thereby betraying our own inner truth. *[Article copies available for a fee from The Haworth Document Delivery Service: 1-800-342-9678. E-mail address:*

Alexander Smith, EdD, ABPP, is a psychologist in Cincinnati, OH. He has been in private practice for 25 years. He has published several papers and chapters on psychotherapy, hypnosis, and more recently on consultation with religious communities. He is completing postgraduate training in the Dynamics of Organizational Consultation Program at the Cincinnati Psychoanalytic Institute. He holds a Diplomate in Counseling Psychology from the American Board of Professional Psychology.

Author note: I wish to thank Abbot John Eudes, OSCO, of Genesee Abbey, NY, and Fr. Matthew Kelty, OSCO, and Br. Patrick Hart, OSCO, of the Abbey of Gethsemani, KY, for their generous reviews of earlier versions of this manuscript and for their balanced perspectives on the life of Thomas Merton. I also wish to thank E. Mark Stern, EdD, ABPP, for his collegial e-mails around the paper itself and on consultation with religious, and Robert Marchesani for his editorial assistance as well as his illuminating comments about religious life.

[Haworth co-indexing entry note]: "Burnt Offerings to Prometheus: The Consultation Meetings Between Thomas Merton and Gregory Zilboorg." Smith, Alexander. Co-published simultaneously in *The Psychotherapy Patient* (The Haworth Press, Inc.) Vol. 11, No. 3/4, 2001, pp. 37-54; and: *Frightful Stages: From the Primitive to the Therapeutic* (ed: Robert B. Marchesani, and E. Mark Stern) The Haworth Press, Inc., 2001, pp. 37-54. Single or multiple copies of this article are available for a fee from The Haworth Document Delivery Service [1-800-342-9678, 9:00 a.m. - 5:00 p.m. (EST). E-mail address: getinfo@ haworthpressinc.com].

KEYWORDS. Restlessness, turmoil, solitude, hermitage, narcissism, ambivalence, authority, discernment, misinterpretation, spirituality, Catholicism

... The truth must dazzle gradually, ere every man be made blind ...

–Emily Dickinson

Even the gods dazzled one another with their brilliance. So went the fateful meetings between the well-known Catholic writer, Thomas Merton, and the prominent figure of American psychiatry, Gregory Zilboorg. Both literary giants were of Promethean origin: on fire and stealing fire, illuminating others in their darkness, redemptive as they transformed their personal sufferings into pages of recognizable faith and hope. Both figures carried in their psyches the dying whimpers of Narcissus: these were the silent cries of unmirrored emptiness, those moments of desolation when even our own images are impoverishing, and when Divine Voices are silent. In their histories, both men sought a state of *aksesis* or the way of spiritual purification: burning off the dross of ego through renunciation, disciplining the senses, and through the transformation of desire in order to attain an experience of God.

But in 1956, the heat was more than either man could bear. In their meetings, Merton and Zilboorg both were blinded by their illusions of the other. They ignored the warnings of Prometheus: that a state of emptiness precedes the fiery metamorphosis of Spirit, and that the idealization of another human is no substitute for the gradual recognition of the Divine truth within. Their story poignantly reminds us that the fire of illumination itself is Divine, belonging to no earthly being. In the end, both Merton and Zilboorg came away burnt by their own greatness.

The force behind these relatively unpublicized consultative meetings at St. John's Abbey in Collegeville, Minnesota, during the summer of 1956 was an Olympic synchronicity: raw, unmediated, and unexpurgated in convergent karma. Thomas Merton was a Trappist monk from the Abbey of Gethsemani in Kentucky. A conversion to Catholicism had transformed his Columbia training as a journalist into a path of haunting self-exploration from France to England to the United States. It culminated in his profession of the monastic life. He recorded his journey in a best seller, *The Seven Story Mountain.* Psychoanalyst Gregory Zilboorg was also a convert to Catholicism, and also from Europe. He too attended Columbia for medical school. Returning to Europe, he trained in psychoanalysis with some of the best-known analysts at the time. He imported a wealth of new ideas to American psychiatry. These coincidents amplify not only the timely fate of their exchanges, but as an event in intellectual history, they exemplified a difficult period of role definitions and uneasy alliance between psychology and the spiritual life.

The meetings appeal to us in many ways. As a human interest story, the meetings deliver a sharp punch, shaking us in our loftiest spiritual aims and luring us into the distracting nitty-gritty of tangled relationships, transferential distortions, and visceral reality. As a professional event, the meetings highlight an inappropriately formed consultation with Zilboorg, later driven by a constellation of unconscious complementary forces in both men. In the study of systems, we have depicted the unique boundary problems that can arise in psychological work with religious communities. The context of the meetings is rich with examples of parallel processes which can flow back and forth between consultants and religious communities, which, left unconscious, become destructive. Most of all, they reveal the pathos within ourselves, in the many roles we play, in the secret alliances we form, and in our needs for ongoing compassion, especially as we struggle at the boundary of psyche and Spirit. They remind us, as the Greek gods did so repeatedly, that our greatest error is that of hubris, of letting our ego presume to be Divine.

AN OVERVIEW OF THE CONSULTATION

The drama of this meeting was contextualized by a surprisingly large supporting cast of influential superiors, friends, colleagues, and fellow monks whose perceptions of psychological consultation at that time would allow these unrealistic expectations within the larger system of religious orders. They are also examples of how vulnerable both consultants and religious can be when naive notions about fraternal charity and obedience turn into rationalized collusions by which one controls another's access to inner freedom.

The meetings were intended to be psychotherapeutic in nature but they did not go well. Archetypal forces materialized into a relationship of dominance and submission, roles well beneath the intellectual stature of each man. In their historical context we learn of Zilboorg's swashbuckling behavior, and of the naive submission by Merton. Yet the driving force of their relationship was a mutually shared fantasy that greatness in another human being is not illusory, and that we need not witness it as a projection of our own grandiosity. The heat created a temporal crucible by which each would relinquish the fantasies of the other, and be plunged into the frozen fire of empty spaces where no image of one's self or another is that much consolation, and where

God can resume working. (The historical summaries cited here are taken from Mott's [1984] biography of Merton, Merton's [1955] recently published "restricted" journal. Zilboorg's writings leave little autobiographical information around these specific events.)

The context for these meetings originates in Merton's growing personal turbulence and in his ongoing authority conflict with Abbot James Fox. The intensity of his conflicts had reached a crisis which some felt necessitated outside intervention. Among other problems between the two was Merton's increased desire to live as a hermit. Merton perceived Fox as too controlling and at times manipulative, never feeling completely supported by Fox. Abbot Fox, perhaps for his own reasons, wanted Merton to receive psychotherapy. When Abbot Fox heard of a conference on psychiatry and the religious life at St. John's Abbey in Collegeville, Minnesota (Benedictine), he pursuaded Merton to attend. Meanwhile, Fox arranged a behind-the-scenes intervention with Abbot Baldwin at St. John's in Collegeville.

The two abbots brought in Gregory Zilboorg, a powerful figure in American psychiatry with a very forceful personality. Ostensibly he was to be a guest speaker, but Fox and Baldwin had the hidden agreement that Zilboorg would work with Merton, even naively hoping that Zilboorg could "analyze" him. The accounts of the meetings, from both Merton and his biographer Mott (1984), indicate that they were conducted in a rather coercive way, leaving Merton feeling at first ambushed and then quite humiliated. The resulting impact upon each figure takes a somewhat surprising twist, with Merton hardening his resistance to Zilboorg's "analysis," and with Zilboorg apparently exposing his own confusing countertransference towards Merton, during which he continued to seek contact with Merton after these meetings, even traveling to Gethsemani.

BACKGROUND OF THE MEETING
FROM MERTON'S PERSPECTIVE

By 1955 Merton had finished his theology studies, having been ordained in 1949. He had now been a Trappist for some fourteen years. The Kentucky monastery named Gethsemani, made popular among World War II veterans following Merton's best-seller, was beginning to burst at the seams with its membership well over two hundred monks. Merton had begun to experience a restlessness with community life. He was haunted by a frustration with the group processes of the community and its leadership. His ambivalence about personalities within the community becomes more clear. As he began to come to terms with his own limits as a monk, he broadened his relationship to a real community of fallible and human brothers. In his intensity as an intellectual, he widened his conceptual reach to understand the growing turmoil within himself about authority, celibacy, and the growing perception that the monastery was not what he had originally imagined. Managing these internal forces exacted a great deal of energy by which he was frequently negatively affected, often in psychosomatic ways.

Several biographical accounts as well as Merton's own journal entries indicate a major shift in his psychological life had taken place in the years following his publication of *Seven Story Mountain.* Merton's honeymoon with the monastery was wearing off, and he now was confronted with the deeper layers of his psyche. His work, *Sign of Jonas,* belies his previously pious and at times sentimental tones and gives us a fresh look at Merton's subjective experience. He began to explore the writings of major spiritual figures of several traditions, both Eastern and Western. At first he began toying with the idea of becoming a Carthusian monk, an order with much more solitude. In later years he would increasingly turn his attention to the East, immersing himself in the studies of Zen, and later Hinduism. Throughout this period he remained committed to his Catholic tradition but with the ever-evolving integration of common connections and themes. In his restlessness, he came to recognize more similarities than differences in experientially defining his own inner truth.

Psychologically, Merton's growing desire for the hermitage seems to have been a symbolic container for many of the unresolved issues that now welled up in the unconscious. He experienced a push within himself to individuate, to think for himself. The pull of old developmental longings was intermingled with a shift in his own understanding of the spiritual life. He was bombarded within by the potential sense of freedom that he intuitively recognized in these studies. Merton's struggle with obedience also seems to have been influenced by a re-emergence of problems of attachments to stable early figures. His mother died when he was six; his father appears to have been somewhat aloof, and to have dealt with depression by frequently changing work and relocating. These events left Merton with a cumulative sense of desertion, highly sensitizing him to issues of separation/individuation, and to struggles with sexuality. Given his intellectual prowess, all of these forces left him frequently shifting between anger and dependency.

Neither Abbot Fox nor Merton recognized how the hermitage had become Merton's symbolic means of a hoped-for resolution, in which he and Fox could co-exist, alone but together. Beyond the potential re-enactments of attachments and losses associated with unresolved parental complexes, the hermitage was also charged with many of the creative forces that drove Merton throughout his life. Through his solitude, he hoped to transcend the limitations of himself and others and, paradoxically, to let his unresolved narcissism transform into more stable perceptions of himself and others.

Merton was struggling personally at this time. His publishing agent, Naomi Burton, was worried about him and saw him as "unsteady." The conflict between solitude and public exposure as a writer was intense and fueled the clash between Merton and Fox, as Fox wanted Merton involved in the community for economic as well as "spiritual" reasons. He had even appointed Merton novice master around this time. By 1955, Merton had begun to explore the applications of psychology to the spiritual life. At that time, within the Church, there was presumably a more intensified ambivalence about the new theories evolving within psychiatry and psychoanalysis. Freudian and neo-Freudian paradigms were a threat to many in the Church, where libido theory, archetypes, and infantile sexuality evoked a paranoid and uninformed reaction. Merton had saturated himself with these issues. He attempted to master complex psychological theories and methods and, without training, apply them as novice master. At times Merton appears to have gone far beyond his training, something that Zilboorg was said to have used as additional ammunition against Merton. For example, Merton administered Rorschach tests to novices who were having emotional difficulties, only later to become confused by organizing the responses, highly complex scoring, and interpretation. Yet, Merton recognized his mistakes and at times his grandiosity. He remained open as an intellectual to potential new meanings and insights that contemporary psychology could offer. He had written a paper entitled "Neurosis in the Monastic Life" and circulated it among colleagues. Later, Zilboorg acquired a copy and would severely criticize its contents as well as Merton himself for his attempt to apply concepts he did not understand. Merton may have actually told Fox about Zilboorg's writings. Mott's (1984) account indicates that Merton later believed that one of the reasons Zilboorg wanted to meet with Merton was to try and prevent him from publishing this paper (Mott, 1984, p. 295). This paper was eventually published in a privately circulated periodical, *Monastic Studies,* by the Benedictines at Mt. Savior Abbey in Elmira, New York (private communication, Stern, 1999).

BACKGROUND OF THE MEETING
FROM ZILBOORG'S PERSPECTIVE

We know relatively little about Zilboorg's subjective experience of Merton. But his biographical foundations, and the papers Zilboorg wrote prior to this meeting, when taken together with the actual behavioral account of the verbal exchange between the two allows some room for interpretation. Yet his background is most impressive.

Zilboorg (1890-1959) was a Russian-born Jew who completed medical corps training in St. Petersburg. He worked at the Psychoneurological Institute there with Bekterev, a major figure in the history of psychology. He participated in the Russian Revolution in 1917, serving as secretary to the minister of labor in the governments of Prince Georgi Lvov and Alexander Kerensky. Following the Bolshevik Revolution, he fled Russia to the United States, where he married. He supported himself through the Columbia University College of Physicians and Surgeons by writing and translating for the theatre. After his graduation and some five years of clinical experience, he attended the Berlin Psychoanalytic Institute, being analyzed by Franz Alexander, a very prominent figure in the Freudian tradition. In 1931, Zilboorg returned to New York and began his psychoanalytic practice.

The next ten years were devoted to the psychoanalytic study of schizophrenic syndromes. He also learned from his patients with post-partum depressions, and theorized an unconscious ambivalence towards motherhood, and sadistic tendencies toward men. He wrote about "ambulatory schizophrenia," a term that now would refer to the borderline personality syndromes. He translated two major works into English: Alexander and Staub's *The Criminal, the Judge and the Public* (1931), and Otto Fenichel's *Outline of Psychoanalysis* (1934).

Zilboorg had a wide range of interests. He is widely noted for his many studies on the history of psychiatry, in particular, *A History of Medical Psychology* (1941). He conceptualized two major shifts in psychiatry. The first was the "pietas literata" or union of service and scholarship. Within this framework he addressed the many works up to the time of Freud. Among these were the writings of Paracelsus, a very interesting and somewhat ironic twist by today's "New Age" standards, where these writings have been re-discovered. In 1941, he published a translation (from Latin) of Paracelsus' *The Diseases That Deprive Man of His Reason.* The second shift was that of Freud's discovery of the unconscious.

Zilboorg's perspective here may gainsay the works of Freud as it seems to ignore the many contributions prior to Freud that were involved in recognizing the unconscious as an influence on human behavior.

An interesting work, often considered his most original contribution, is *The Medical Man and the Witch During the Renaissance* (1935). This work reviewed the malevolent attitudes toward women existent within the *Malleus Maleficarium* (1486) which had served as a reference text for the prosecution of alleged witches. Zilboorg sought, through the reinterpretation of behavior and motives, to minimize the role of demonic influences and to reconceptualize them as originating within the psyche as projected unwanted aspects of the self.

By 1944, Zilboorg had well established himself as a figure within psychoanalysis and psychiatry. He served as an associate editor of *One Hundred Years of American Psychiatry.* He was a co-founder of *Psychoanalytic Quarterly.* In 1954 he published *The Psychology of the Criminal Act and Punish-*

ment. This was a body of lectures delivered at Yale in which he called for the evaluation of the total personality of the criminal, and questioned the unconscious motivations of judges.

Zilboorg's papers on the psychological aspects of spirituality suggest more than a passing interest about eremitical life, asceticism, and the intense struggle between the instinctual drives and the monastic ideal. They reflect the writing style within psychoanalysis at the time in which new paradigms about the vicissitudes of instinctual life are considered against the Freudian conceptual standard. Some of these essays attempt to recontextualize the course of love as a spiritual transformation of instinct. Zilboorg also recognized the potentials and blocks within psychological life for meaningful spiritual attainment. However, his writing seems to omit the intervention of grace, leaving with spiritual attainment the solipsistic quality of "self-control" as the principal means to union with God.

Zilboorg's ambivalence towards the authority of Freud provides an interesting parallel to that of Merton's struggle with Abbot Fox about the hermitage. Zilboorg omitted considering the broader revisions of psychoanalysis that had been directly applied to the spiritual life, such as the works of Jung. Zilboorg's own need for control may well reflect a conflict about emancipating himself from his own training. It also appears to have influenced his understanding of the spiritual life. He seems to have struggled with his own ambivalence about orthodox psychoanalysis. He attempted to extract essential principles from the Freudian model, at times wanting to speak the party line, and at other times recognizing the need to challenge the orthodox thinking on love as it exists in the spiritual life. In this way, he avoided the reductive stance of psychoanalytic orthodoxy that essentially views the longing for union with God as a regressive wish to return to early mothering experiences.

It is interesting to review Zilboorg's essay on "A Psychiatric Consideration of the Ascetical Ideal" (in Stone-Zilboorg, 1962). He addresses the issue of suffering, distinguishing the dissolution of ego-bound desire from masochism:

> ... suffering is masochism only when it is a perversion, when it leads directly to sexual gratification or when it is a singular substitute for it. ...
> (Zilboorg, 1962, p. 69)

In this same essay, he addresses the issue of power of others as an unconscious influence. His comments may well apply to himself:

> (Such) unconscious hostility makes a man live in the forces which give him a sense of power over others. This sense of power may be expressed in many ways: for instance through the acquisition of unneces-

sary wealth, or through a sense of which thwarts a man's rational desire
to exert his will in the direction of object-libidinous interest and instead
evolves in him the captious, impulsive, yet persevering all powerful
egocentricity which gives illusions of great will power. (Zilboorg,
1962, pp. 70-71)

Psychoanalytic theory had not developed the currently understood types of
narcissistic disorders, nor their potential for transformation and growth. At
the time of his writing, Zilboorg's thinking therefore could not address by
today's standards the healing of self-alienation, fragmentation, and emptiness
as Merton seems to have experienced them. Zilboorg's clarification of neurosis within spirituality, however, remains relevant for contemporary religious
life. He gives a context for understanding the aims of ascetical love as being
on the one hand bound by the total constellation of man's basic instincts, and
on the other by the superordinate "caritas and agape." According to Zilboorg, the realization of these ascetic ideals presumes a level of mature
psychosocial development in which the neurotic struggles have been re-
solved.

When Zilboorg's writings about the spiritual life and his reported behavior
with Merton are taken together as a whole, one can get the impression that
Zilboorg at times may have wished he could trade places with Merton. There
is a restless quality to Zilboorg's spiritually oriented essays, one that can
leave the reader with a sense that Zilboorg is "not quite" or "almost" grasping commonly recognized principles such as ego surrender, the "dark night,"
union with God. Zilboorg's greatest strength, i.e., his understanding of the
unconscious forces that affect one's motivation, discernment, and inner truth,
is also his greatest limitation in that he remains bound to his paradigm of
humanly directed spiritual attainment. At the very least, Zilboorg appears to
have been disturbed by Merton's interest in the eremitical life, perhaps even
envious of Merton's blend of monastic life and reputation as a writer and
monk. As discussed below, Zilboorg took particular aim at Merton's most
vulnerable spot, accusing him of wanting "a hermitage in Times Square with
a sign over it saying 'HERMIT'" (Mott, 1984, p. 297).

ABBOT FOX'S PERSPECTIVE
ABOUT THE CONSULTATION PROCESS

Merton's biographers vary in their kindness towards Abbot Fox's motives
about Merton. A somewhat controversial figure himself, Fox has been seen by
some as caring about Merton yet also frankly concerned about the revenue
generated by the royalties from Merton's writings. Indeed Fox himself was a
graduate of the Harvard School of Business who had taken over his abbatial

duties when Gethsemani was having significant financial problems. It is to his credit that the abbey was able to re-establish its financial well-being during his tenure. Leaving aside for the moment his own transferential distortions about Merton, Abbot Fox appears to have had an unrealistic idea about consultation itself, one that Zilboorg would basically "fix" Merton. Fox's motives about intervening probably ranged from the abbatial concerns for the well-being of one of his monks to the more practical concerns for the monastic community.

On the balance, Abbot Fox appears to have met his match with his responsibilities to Merton. More recent biographical accounts support a more compassionate view of both as rather complicated men who could not understand their relationship to each other. A most recent discussion of Fox's tenure as abbot views him in more humane and less entrepreneurial terms than many of the earlier ones that may have overidentified with Merton's perspective (Aprile, 1998). Monks who lived with Merton see Abbot Fox as having had his hands full managing Merton's temperament and often insatiable intellect. Despite an often-cited view that Fox was exploiting Merton's literary talents for the economic good of the monastery, Abbot Fox clearly had Merton's well-being in mind (Bamberger, 1998). An ironic twist to the saga about the hermitage is that Fox himself aspired to seeking the greater solitude of a hermitage, but due to the prevailing Trappist rule at the time, he could not permit himself this pursuit until the years following his retirement as abbot (Kelty, 1999). (Abbot Fox and Thomas Merton now lie buried next to each other in the abbey cemetery.)

These considerations contrast restrospectively with the transferential distortions Fox appears to have formed about Merton at the time, leaving him unable to objectify Merton simply as a monk who was having trouble with aspects of his calling. Fox seems to have "taken the bait" from Merton just as Merton would similarly be provoked by Fox. As a superior, Fox appears to have been unable to detach from Merton's emotional turmoil. The power struggle that developed from Fox's perspective seems to have fueled his own need for control of Merton, whose issues easily complemented those of Fox. The hermitage and Merton's deepening interest in solitude may have affronted Fox's own investment in interpreting Cistercian rule, and in his apparent over-identification with the authority. Merton seems to have become an embarrassment to Fox's competence both as a spiritual leader and as a superior. Fox's own need to go to such lengths as engineering Zilboorg's visit suggests that the resolution of Merton's difficulty became his own obsession, a measure of his own self-esteem and effectiveness as a superior.

THE MEETING BETWEEN MERTON AND ZILBOORG

Mott's (1984) account of the context for this meeting indicates that from several perspectives Zilboorg had a strong personal interest in "treating"

Merton. Robert Giroux at Harcourt Brace, a personal friend and publisher of both Merton and Zilboorg, had suggested that the two meet. Merton was reading the works of Karen Horney and some commentaries on Jung. He himself enthusiastically supplied Zilboorg with a copy of "Neurosis in the Monastic Life" through Giroux. Zilboorg was known to have been anxious to meet Merton. At this same time, Abbot Fox was arranging with Abbot Baldwin that Merton and Fr. John Eudes Bamberger would be in attendance at the conference at St. John's Abbey. Giroux was concerned that Zilboorg seemed to have preconceptions about Merton even before meeting. Counter-balancing this view is one that Giroux himself may have been more involved with arranging the meetings than previously thought, and that Zilboorg's eagerness may have been in part due to the promptings of Merton's friends (Hart, 1999).

In New York, Zilboorg said that he had already analyzed Merton from his writing and felt confident that he knew what the trouble was. Giroux interpreted Zilboorg's wish to help as laced with rivalry. Zilboorg wrote a letter to Merton dated June 6, 1956. Mott's analysis suggests that there was a sarcastic quality, perhaps with a patronizing tone in Zilboorg's letter. Zilboorg advised Merton to begin reading Karl Abraham rather than Freud. This is an interesting twist for two reasons in that Abraham's main works are on depression, and Abraham himself was a close student of Freud.

Mott suggests that Zilboorg himself was in "no state of objectivity" when at St. John's (Mott, 1984, p. 292), and that although it was true that Merton had crossed professional lines in his role as novice master, that this gave Zilboorg "further ammunition" to assume the upper hand with Merton. Mott's generous interpretation is that Zilboorg's main concern was to "deal with somebody he regarded as a quack" (Mott, 1984, p. 292). Mott also indicates that Zilboorg viewed Merton's paper ("Neurosis and Monastic Life") as "academic poaching" (Mott, 1984, p. 291) and suggests that Zilboorg's overt worry–that publishing the paper could harm Merton's reputation–was, in common psychoanalytic parlance, a "reaction formation," i.e., doing the opposite of the forbidden impulse. In this way, Giroux perhaps sensed that Zilboorg was expressing a muted envy about Merton by assuming an unsolicitied "helpful" (but hostile) approach. Zilboorg, according to Merton's journals, went on to criticize the article as "utterly inadequate, hastily written, should not even be revised . . ." (Mott, 1984, p. 294).

During the conference, Merton's first encounter with Zilboorg took the form of a question as a member of the audience. Merton asked Zilboorg, "How do you define the dysfunction of a neurotic?" Zilboorg is said to have stared at Merton for several seconds and then said, ". . . science does not start with a definition but ends with it." Fr. John Eudes reported noticing this glaring behavior on Zilboorg's part towards Merton when Merton had discussed Zen with Dr. Howard Phillips Rome, another lecturer.

The first private conference with Zilboorg occurred on July 29, 1956. Mott provides a synopsis of Merton's "restricted journal" entries which only recently have been made public. Merton's entries indicate that Zilboorg "engineered" Merton's attendance through Abbot Baldwin, out of concern for the article being published and about Merton's well-being. Merton perceived Zilboorg as "accusing" him of being a neurotic, of being "dependent" on words, of being a "gadfly to your superiors," of being very stubborn and of being "afraid to be an ordinary monk in the community."

Merton's entries go on to reveal Zilboorg's accusatory tone taking on almost abusive proportions. Zilboorg told Merton that he and Fr. John Eudes could easily become a pair of "semi-psychotic quacks." Zilboorg then presumes to read Merton's mind, stating that in his talk with Dr. Rome, Merton thought only of himself and wanted to use Dr. Rome for his own aggrandizement, and that he thought nothing of his priesthood, the apostolate, the Church or his soul. Merton quotes Zilboorg as claiming that he

> . . . likes to be famous, (you) want to be a big shot, you keep pushing your way out–into publicity–megalomania and narcissism are your big trends . . . (your) hermit trend is pathological . . . these are not things you can foresee, they are traps you fall into as you go along . . . it is not intelligence you lack but affectivity. . . . [suggesting that Merton intellectualized as a defense against experiencing feeling states] (Mott, 1984, pp. 295-296)

Of some concern and interest is Mott's rather disturbing note that Zilboorg then instructed Merton not to speak to anyone about their conversation. Merton's first reactions include a range of negative and positive emotion. The following day he wrote to Naomi Burton, his publishing agent, that Zilboorg had been "terrific," and that he was the first to really understand what Merton's struggles were about. Mott indicates that when Abbot Fox arrived for the conference, Merton had genuine cause for concern about Zilboorg creating any "evidence" that Merton was unstable. Fox had written to Cardinal Montini (later Pope Paul VI) in May of 1955 implying that Merton was temperamental, and too artistically volatile for his own spiritual good. Fox had quoted from a letter written by Fr. Barnabas Mary Ahern dated January 29, 1953 to Merton. In it, Fr. Barnabas warned Merton that any departure from Gethsemani would undermine Merton's growing public identification with the abbey and the contributions of his writing. It is not clear how Fox came to quote the letter to Cardinal Montini except through the then-practiced censuring of mail to the monastery. Abbot Fox then appeared to be looking for reasons to justify his "grounding" of Merton's interests in becoming a hermit. Merton was now put in the position of having to demonstrate an emotional stability while enduring the provocation of Zilboorg's 'analysis' and Abbot Fox's judgment of his artistic restlessness.

The story then takes a more difficult turn for Merton. Zilboorg himself called for a second conference. Mott's narrative painfully stands by itself:

> In these circumstances it was very unfortunate that Zilboorg called a second conference and discussed the "case" of Father Louis in the presence of his abbot. At the second interview Gregory Zilboorg stuck to the question of Merton's religious vocation and his life as a monk, a would-be hermit. He seems to have started off affably enough, taking a "Well, what are we going to do about this?" line of approach. Merton was not ready to be exposed in front of Dom James (Fox). He flew into a fury and cried tears of rage. For Merton's abbot there had been no preparation, no preliminary interview. . . . Zilboorg went on repeating in a level voice what he had said before about the hermitage idea being pathological: "You want a hermitage in Times Square with a large sign over it saying 'HERMIT.'" This time one's sympathy is entirely with Merton, who saw himself trapped, and who sat with tears streaming down his face muttering "Stalin! Stalin!" The worst thing that could have happened had happened: Zilboorg had told him to tell nobody, then he staged a situation in which the most exaggerated misgivings of Dom James were dramatically confirmed. . . . These were the most damaging ten minutes since he (Merton) had left the world for the monastery. (Mott, 1984, p. 297)

In the context of the Promethean myth, this exchange between Merton and Zilboorg was ill-fated from the beginning. The underlying dynamics do not begin with unconscious envy, nor with the need to idealize another, though arguably these motives exerted enormous force as well. Instead, the context of the story itself is about a subtle but frequent shift in perspective when mental health consultants attempt to work with matters of spirituality. The change in perspective seems to occur unconsciously, from understanding the psyche within the context of spirituality to presuming to interpret the work of Spirit within the psychic life. The difference in approach, one to which both Merton and Zilboorg colluded, squarely placed them both in the untenable position of doing the work of the gods, of presuming to let the interpretive powers of psychoanalysis have an illuminative freedom that was not its own. Spiritual illumination itself was the symbolic redemption of Prometheus given to humanity, one that must burn as it enlightens–slowly.

The Promethean context makes the story all the more painful to read. One can only begin to imagine the tensions that broke forth among all three participants. Each figure clearly distorted the other. A strange cadence of projected images flowed among the three figures. Merton appears to have viewed the renowned psychoanalyst Zilboorg in largely idealizing ways until he felt torpedoed. Zilboorg in turn seems to have been driven by a complicated mix of possible envy, needs for admiration and power, and possible projections of himself into Merton. Zilboorg was unable to recognize these problems within both himself and Merton. It is not clear how Abbot Fox came to view Zilboorg at this point. It would seem that his "calling in the cavalry" played right into Zilboorg's grandiosity and hidden agendas.

UNCONSCIOUS INTERACTIONS
AND THE CONSULTATION CONTRACT

The account leaves the reader stunned, wondering how the well-meaning consultation could result in such a chilling misuse of its purpose. Any consensus among modern-day superiors would most likely recognize the boundary violations among all parties, the loss of distance on the part of Zilboorg, the tacit complicity on the part of Merton's superiors, and Merton's own contributions to the existing conflict around authority.

From a systems point of view, as the contract was arranged, Zilboorg worked for Abbot Fox, and not for Merton. Yet all parties succumbed to the subtle shift in perception that Zilboorg was "treating" Merton. Zilboorg proceeded unchallenged to presume to do both, i.e., to work for Abbot Fox and to designate Merton as "the patient." No mention is made of the inherent conflict of interest on Zilboorg's part. Further, none of the parties questioned the appropriateness of such an alliance, nor recognized that these meetings under these conditions would be a departure from the usual confidentiality. Instead, Zilboorg, Merton, and Fox all appear to have been mesmerized by a misinterpretation of the vow of obedience, and together dispensed with the ordinary boundaries that would protect all involved. No clarification of the contract occurred that allowed it to be recognized as an agreement. Rather, under the guise of charity, all three unconsciously colluded to search for a miraculous cure for Merton's problem. Zilboorg's state of mind allowed him to presume that he indeed had such a cure. Zilboorg's greatest mistake is that he kept Merton as the "patient" and failed to take into account the relationship conflict between Merton and Abbot Fox.

The meetings between Merton and Zilboorg dramatically illustrate that there are unconscious interactions between the consultant and the individual or system which exert a defining force in the consultative process. At the very least Zilboorg presumed to enter into a relationship to which Merton had not fully agreed nor about which he was fully informed. Zilboorg appears to have been a victim of his own grandiosity in that he communicated a highly patronizing and "infallible" presence to the conditions of the consultation.

This behavior in turn exerted enormous pressure on Merton. As stated earlier, these same attitudes and behavior were also disabling to Abbot Fox. The outcome of the meeting also essentially thwarted Abbot Fox's needs to em-power himself with any improved method of dealing with Merton. They removed from Fox's grasp the very tools he sought but which he could not verbalize: namely, an operational understanding and a way of dealing with Merton's difficulties in solvable terms.

Zilboorg's lack of stated clarity about whose problem was being addressed further added to the confusion. As reported, Zilboorg never appears clear in identifying that he was trying to assist Abbot Fox in dealing with Merton. Abbot Fox's needs are never really defined in consultative terms at all. Yet Zilboorg's employer was Abbot Fox. This confusion probably reflects as-pects of psychological consultation that were not yet developed at that time and which easily gave Zilboorg greater opportunity to get lost in the highly charged issues of the moment. Zilboorg appears to have played out a relation-ship in which he identified with the idealizing projections of both Fox and Merton. He then splits Merton and Fox, casting himself as an interpreter of Merton's psyche to Abbot Fox. He then goes a step further and devalues and humiliates Merton. We do not know his internal reasons for doing so, but it does seem quite plausible that Zilboorg was defending himself against ad-miration and/or envy. Zilboorg appears over-taken by his own aggression, overwhelmed, having lost his capacity for objectivity and professional dis-tance. Instead he created a dominant/submissive relational tone which later shut down Merton to future contacts.

UNDERSTANDING CREATIVE SPACE
IN CONSULTATION WITH RELIGIOUS

Consultation with religious brings into play a unique constellation of private experiences which form a background against which an individual or a group copes with some issue or problem. By its nature, this context always has in it the spiritual life as it continues to evolve. Regardless of specific training, traditions and customs, whatever unresolved developmental prob-lems, neurotic anxieties, and inhibitions that may have emerged in the identi-fiable form, they are always juxtaposed to a most private and vulnerable aspect of the individual religious here understood as creative space. When the consultant does not recognize and protect the consultee's creative space as an experiential sanctuary, both consultant and consultee easily polarize into a complementarity of distortions about each another, i.e., savior/sinner, or om-nipotent knower/ignorant fool, or lifeguard/drowning man.

Creative space is a term used by the well-known British psychoanalyst D. W. Winnicott. In adult life, it refers to an experientially defined aspect of ourselves in which our conscious awareness is neither located in internal fantasy, nor bound by the perceptual demands of our outer realities. Creative space is essentially a "third area" (Winnicott, 1971) that requires no commitment to forms of learning, however we cognitively represent them, nor is it defined by the streams of spontaneous reverie. Coppolillo (1976) refers to this area of experience as a "zone of optimal control" in which we are as far as we need to be from both the press of external reality demands as well as from our own internal stimuli. Bollas (1992) describes how living only in the objective world, without entering this third area, essentially blunts the evocative-transformational aspects of our relationship to outer reality (and God?) and leaves us experientially constricted, reality bound, and barren. We become like children who cannot play.

Recognizing the role of creative space provides this "temenos" or protective internal shelter where the individual may be alone in relation to God, not as a prescribed experience but as an ongoing process of discovery. This is not a matter of technique since by definition there is no technique to produce creative space. Thus old and new, internal and external have their say without impinging, pressuring, cajoling, or draining the individual because someone said so. The experience of God can become progressively free of misleading notions, letting the experience of God be filtered through moments of an "unthought known" (Bollas, 1991).

The concept of creative space bridges the consultant's psychological orientation to the spiritual experience of the consultee without impinging upon it. The manner in which consultation issues and problems are addressed must take into account the individual's own spiritual process as it continues to be formed. The consultee grapples with an identified problem but in the context of ongoing perceptual shifts and clarifications that arise in the spiritual life. The consultant therefore must externally honor the internal process of the consultee by recognizing that there is an experiential dimension which is not his/her business to attempt to modify or influence, or at times even to understand. The consultant must make room for this relationship to God which s/he may not ever fully comprehend but which s/he must nonetheless protect. Caplan (1972) usefully describes these non-intrusive methods of consultation with clergy:

> Consultation, therefore, takes a safer, more economical route, and one that is more dignified for the consultee. Instead of stripping away the defenses of the personality in order to dig out unconscious material, consultation tries to strengthen these defenses, shore up the ego at its weaker points, and enable the individual to function better and more comfortably, even though he, like most of humanity, might never be a paragon of mental health and maturity . . . the effectiveness of consultation depends, paradoxically, precisely on the consultant's recognition

and identification, *though never his explicit mention,* of the emotional entanglement of the minister with his case. (Caplan, 1972, p. 51)

Zilboorg could not recognize Merton's conflict in positive terms. He could not view the need for the hermitage as Merton's use of potential space, that it had a creative significance for his own psychological development, nor that it was part of a larger process that could take Merton beyond his ego. Zilboorg's attack on Merton's ego suggests that he could not empathically tolerate the emptiness that such moments can carry. Merton, for his own part, later demonstrated a resiliency and capacity for distancing himself from all that was so highly charged. He was able to see Zilboorg in more compassionate and even-handed terms.

From a bird's eye view, it is curious–some would say karmic–that Zilboorg and Merton should wind up meeting under such circumstances. There is a quality of fate or destiny that their paths converged, one for which we can in many ways be grateful. To be sure, one cannot ignore the consciously experienced intentions of Fox, Merton, and Zilboorg. Each wanted something good to come of the consultation. It is indeed ironic that these established intellectuals, powerful and influential in their respective fields, could not reflect their respective strengths and capabilities in these meetings. In the nexus of it all lie three very large egos, all longing for an experience of God and each caught in his own unconscious pull towards untransformed narcissism. As egos they became burnt offerings to Prometheus, torchbearers that illuminate our way a little further. The meetings teach us to be cautious about consultations with spiritual matters, reminding us that the spiritual life easily constellates unmediated complexes with powerfully inflating energies. These energies themselves crackle with the compassionate light of Prometheus when we can let him hold the light for us.

REFERENCES

Aprile, D. (1998). *The Abbey of Gethsemani: place of peace and paradox.* Louisville: Trout Lily Press.
Bamberger, Fr. John Eudes. (1998) Personal communication, April 14th.
Bollas, C. (1991). *Being a character: psychoanalyses and self experience.* New York: Hill and Wang.
Braceland, F.J. (1960). In memoriam: Gregory Zilboorg. *American J. of Psychiatry,* 116, 671-672.
Caplan, R. (1972). *Helping the helpers to help.* New York: Seabury Press.
Coppolillo, H. (1976). The transitional phenomenon resisted. *American Journal of Child & Adolescent Psychiatry,* 15, 36-48.
Cunningham, L.S. ed. (1997). *A search for solitude: the journals of Thomas Merton Vol 3 1952-1960,* San Francisco: Harper.

Hart, Br. Patrick. (1999). Personal communication. Abbey of Gethsemani.

Kelty, Fr. Matthew (1999). Personal communication. Abbey of Gethsemani.

Merton, T. (1953). *The sign of Jonas.* New York: Harcourt, Brace and Co.

Mott, M. (1984). *The seven mountains of Thomas Merton.* New York: Houghton Mifflin Co.

Winnicott, D.W. (1971). *Playing and reality.* London: Tavistock.

Zilboorg, G. (1928). Postpartum schizophrenias. *J of Nervous and Mental Diseases,* 68, 370-383.

_____ (1935). *The medical man and the witch during the renaissance.* New York: Cooper Square Publishing.

_____ (1941). *Sigmund Freud: his exploration of the mind of man.* New York: Scribners.

_____ (1941). *A history of medical psychology.* New York: W.W. Norton.

_____ (1954). *The psychology of the criminal act and punishment.* New York: Harcourt, Brace.

_____ (1962). A psychiatric consideration of the ascetic ideal. In M. Stone-Zilboorg (ed.) *Psychoanalysis and Religion.* New York: Farrar, Strauss & Cudahy.

The Nights and Knights of Cabiria: Modern Woman in Search of Her Soul

Edward Mendelowitz

SUMMARY. This is an essay about quest and emotion and what we may call the metaphorically feminine. These aspects of existence are, in my mind, inextricably linked and relate in the end to nature, interiority, and even love: a non-parochial politic and unfolding of soul. Cabiria's journey toward self and divinity takes place far beyond system or church and points the way toward that which each of us must undertake if we are to find ourselves in the world and chaos we live in. It is the stuff of psychotherapy besides. What Cabiria attains is poignant and precious and yet, in its very profundity, difficult to articulate or define. A knowing smile and unforgettable glance at the camera eye at the close of our film says it all. Have we perhaps cheapened psychology by submitting it to a kind of fanatical algorithm and reduction? Have we perhaps trivialized paradise by construing it as overly concrete and literal, thereby casting it blithely into the stratosphere?

Like all great works of art, Fellini's *Nights of Cabiria* may be considered from multiple positions and steadfastly resists the neat analyses of

---

Edward Mendelowitz did his doctoral work at the California School of Professional Psychology in Berkeley, where he worked closely with Rollo May. He is in private practice in Lexington, Massachusetts, and on the faculty of the Film and Psychology Series at the Boston Institute of Psychotherapy. He has presented papers at recent APA conferences on individuation and Oedipus, film and modernity, and ethics and eastern thought, and on the work of the playwright Pirandello at the European Congress of Psychology last year in Rome. Ed is a contributing author to Schneider and May's *Psychology of Existence* and Jim Bugental et al.'s forthcoming *Handbook of Humanistic Psychology*. His writing and talks attempt to get to the heart of the humanistic, existential, esthetical, and even spiritual bases of our field in their evocation of imagination, transience, possibility, and awe.

[Haworth co-indexing entry note]: "The Nights and Knights of Cabiria: Modern Woman in Search of Her Soul." Mendelowitz, Edward. Co-published simultaneously in *The Psychotherapy Patient* (The Haworth Press, Inc.) Vol. 11, No. 3/4, 2001, pp. 55-91; and: *Frightful Stages: From the Primitive to the Therapeutic* (ed: E. Mark Stern, and Robert B. Marchesani) The Haworth Press, Inc., 2001, pp. 55-91. Single or multiple copies of this article are available for a fee from The Haworth Document Delivery Service [1-800-342-9678, 9:00 a.m. - 5:00 p.m. (EST). E-mail address: getinfo@haworthpressinc.com].

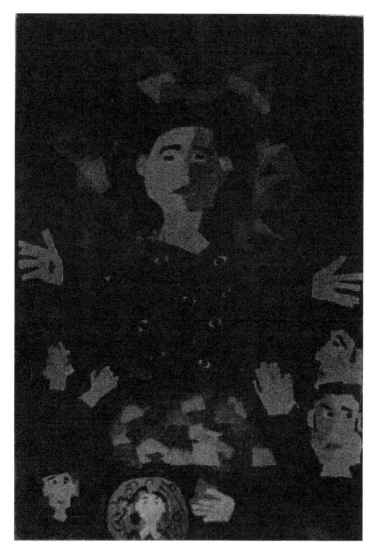

The reproduction of the painting which serves as our frontispiece was made by a patient of mine. Kristiana's haunting *God Mother* suggests some of the agony and puzzlement and sheer terror of existence no less than a prayer for passage, patronage, and sanctuary. It recalls (through its depiction of austerity and inwardness, passion and nuance, fragmentation reconciled briefly through color and form) many of the themes which Fellini himself is about. It is to this patient, a young woman who embodies all the spontaneity and pain and humor and compassion of Cabiria, to whom this essay is dedicated. This is done with what Medard Boss had called "therapeutic eros," with gratitude for what therapists learn from patients who subsist along margins and yet may well possess fortitudes and insights which we professionals too often lack. It should come as no surprise that Fellini's imaginative vision was imbued with surpassing sympathy for what he had called "poetic lunacy" and inspired a body of work which manifests uncanny feeling for "the individuality of eccentricity." "It seems to me," he tells Charlotte Chandler in her heartfelt *I, Fellini*, "that sanity is learning to tolerate the intolerable, to go on without screaming." I cannot help thinking that patient and filmmaker would have understood each other. Certainly, each has much to teach us and say. (Painting reproduced by permission of artist.)

guilds, academies, and experts. It is likely that Fellini would have fa-
vored this more poetical rendering over the standard clinical fare.
Clearly the film has much to do with trial and loss, perseverance and
sham, and a woman's ultimate recovery of her own inner resources. We
may think about the Christ story as we consider this essay, about the
Stations of the Cross and the age-old biblical theme of growth through
suffering. See if you do not discern a sort of gnostic reworking of our
commoner notions about death and resurrection, ignorance and light,
love in both these realms and those. Contemplating our caseloads and
disciplines and our own lives as well, we begin to see that our text is
universal in its evocation and calling, its creator always meditating on
the beauty and travesty of things and the possibilities which inhere in a
more genuine life, one which beholds the mystery and design with awe
and obeisance and proceeds with humility and grace. *[Article copies available for a fee from The Haworth Document Delivery Service: 1-800-342-9678.
E-mail address: <getinfo@haworthpressinc.com> Website: <http://www.
HaworthPress.com> © 2001 by The Haworth Press, Inc. All rights reserved.]*

KEYWORDS. Fellini, poetry, filmmakers, consciousness, humiliation,
misfortune, mindfulness, inauthenticity, discernment, ascendance, me-
tanoia, awakening, psychoanalysis, Italy, renewal

And opening my eyes, I am afraid of course
to look–this inward look that society scorns.
Still, I search in these woods and find nothing worse
than myself, caught between the grapes and the thorns.

–Anne Sexton
Kind Sir: These Woods

For Kristiana,

For nothing can be sole or whole
That has not been rent.

–W. B. Yeats
Crazy Jane Talks with the Bishop

Change my life! Grant my prayer, too. Help me change my life!

–Cabiria (kissing the ground before the image
of the Holy Mother at *Madonna del Divino Amore*)

"How should we live?" someone asked me in a letter.
I had meant to ask him the same question.

Again, and as ever,
as may be seen above,
the most pressing questions
are naïve ones.

-Wislawa Szymborska
The Century's Decline

[The creator], becoming arrogant in spirit, boasted himself over all those things that were below him and exclaimed, "I am father and God, and above me there is no other." But his mother, hearing him speak thus, cried out against him, "Do not lie, Ialdaboath."

-Iranaeus
Libros Quinque Adversus Haereses

The living spirit grows and even outgrows its earlier forms of expression; it freely chooses the [women and] men in whom it lives and who proclaim it. This living spirit is eternally renewed and pursues its goal in manifold and inconceivable ways throughout the history of [human]kind. Measured against it, the names and forms which [we] have given it mean little enough; they are only the changing leaves and blossoms on the stem of the eternal tree.

-C. G. Jung
Modern Man in Search of a Soul

I have felt the swaying of the elephant's shoulders, and now you want me to climb on a jackass? Try to be serious.

-Mirabai
Why Mira Can't Go Back to Her Old House

Among the filmmakers whose work both merits perennial admiration and scrutiny as art and is of a fundamentally psychological cast, Federico Fellini is the one to whom I find myself most eternally returned. It is through some diabolical admixture of native intelligence, reverential awareness, Italian intuition, and narrative pathos and lyricism that the filmmaker attains his utterly unique perspective and brilliance. Fellini hits, truly, on all cylinders, an accomplishment which had earned for him, almost from the beginning, the accolade of having been a poet in whom we might have absolute faith.[1] He is auteur par excellence, one with humanitarian large-heartedness and uncanny humor and postmodern nostalgia which can put the academic, in her or his typical sterility, to shame. Through an abiding belief in the story at hand and the power of imagination to inform, the director illumines the fundamental human themes and, as any artist must, gives voice to his distinct variation on these themes in the process. What is life, after all, if not a theme with variations?

One of the abiding themes in Fellini's work is the relationship between the sexes: the commodification of women by men through the pursuit of a sexualized holy grail of femininity and thereby the longed-for bliss of completeness and union, fleeting freedom from thought and anxiety and self-consciousness. Yet beneath the compulsivity of sexual conquest and release which informs the artist's psychic landscape we find, inexorably, the far more subtle yearning for genuine, unadulterated human encounter. The truer jewel lies further beyond and within. The director himself (in Keel and Strich, 1976, p. 61) articulates his ulterior motive and lodestone:

> Our trouble, as modern[s], is loneliness, and this begins in the very depths of our being. No public celebration or political symphony can hope to be rid of it. Only between man and man[2] . . . can this solitude be broken, only through individual people can a kind of message be passed, making [us] understand–almost *discover*–the profound link between one person and the next.

More enamored of Jung than Freud, it is to Fellini's credit that he remains nonetheless true to his own sensibility and calling (what Buber had called one's "particular way") in the end, thereby attaining an insight and grace and body of work that perhaps neither theorist was quite able to match or sustain.[3] It was the psychoanalytic misfit Otto Rank who had foreseen already in the thirties that film might one day succeed in shedding light on psychological nuance where the printed word would and could not.

Fellini manifests psychoanalytic and–more than this–psychospiritual perspicacity in placing the quest for the feminine (what he had called the "poetry of woman" or "feminine affectiveness") at the center of many of his films while understanding full well that what is ultimately desired lies beyond and beneath the simply sexual: more mysterious still and yet more difficult to define or maintain and, even when glimpsed or received, humanly temporal. The director, who liked to joke about not having read Proust or Joyce or whomever when the critics made grandiloquent claims about the influence of such writers on his work,[4] nonetheless knew wherefrom to take his cues and was inspired throughout his life and career[5] by his wife and most memorable actress, the inimitable and, indeed, startling Giulietta Masina. "Giulietta is a special case," Fellini (ibid., p. 105), had said, "the true soul" and "inspiration" of films for which "she herself is the theme."

The film we consider here is *The Nights of Cabiria* (1956), made just two years after the triumph of *La Strada* (1954), Fellini's first patent masterpiece. Masina plays the part of a common prostitute who seeks unwitting transcendence of an everyday world of power, manipulation, seduction, and charade. We may think of it as a woman's film which focuses on the heroine's extrication from a world of male domination and influence, though we are wise to think along other lines as well. Digging a bit deeper we discern, at the furthermost reaches of inquiry, a universal work about the very human quest for salvation and meaning and love. *The Nights of Cabiria* documents at last the irrepressible longing for something beyond what is given and had, the desire, as William James had said, for something "more." It is an impulse and passion that dwells in all.[6] As such our film coexists both at the point of and also beyond dichotomy and politics, thereby propelling itself far above prosaic psychologies and voguish movements and books so blithely championed by proponents of the new and fashionable.

It seems to be at least one half of an enduring truth that nothing important is easily won. Fellini seems to have grasped this fact implicitly as well: his films rarely end on the joyous note.[7] He is an old pro after all, "a psychologist," as the philosopher Nietzsche had once said of himself, "with ears even behind ears." Nietzsche was speaking metaphorically, of course, as facile minds tend and prefer to do, but Fellini literally had eyes (his own) behind eyes (the camera's) and knew it. In the service of genius, such vision becomes, truly, the "Eye of Shiva," the insight of gods and vision of saints with director and artist as arbiter and guide. What better vehicle, then, to shed light on the vagaries of life and yearnings of the human spirit and soul? Let us open our eyes and ears and, yes, even our hearts and contemplate a work of psychological and spiritual mastery.

On the outskirts of Rome the prostitute Cabiria is strolling playfully with Georgio, the new man in her life. We see her from a distance, a body devoid of face or individuality, happily deluded in her state of romantic intrigue and ignorance. Within moments she is at the edge of the Tiber, Georgio beside her, as she swings her purse flamboyantly through the air. Georgio looks about furtively and–seeing that they are alone–snatches the purse, pushes Cabiria into the river, and disappears into the day and the city. Not knowing how to swim, our heroine sinks like a stone. A boy appears from behind some shrubbery and shouts. (*"It's a woman. There she is!"*) Other boys appear almost out of nowhere and dive in to rescue this pathetic waif.

Laid prostrate by the banks of the river, Cabiria is quickly surrounded by men and boys who have gathered at the spectacle and now restore her to everyday consciousness and life. Throughout is the plainsong of Italian machismo: "We saved her," one boy proudly proclaims. "We rescued her!" She went under "three times" another exclaims, thereby calling attention to the implied baptism that has just taken place. Even a man who would humbly defer good works and outcomes to other beings and realms casts his metaphysical allusions in predictably masculine garb: *"You can thank the Holy Father."* But Cabiria, having regained colloquial consciousness, has little use for an anonymous patronage and chauvinism[8] with which she is all too well acquainted. She thinks of only one man (one who has just tried to bring about her demise and yet whom, through the near-universal proclivity to the transference implied in quotidian relations,[9] she had taken for more noble substance and stock) as she now kicks a boy who tries to assist the others in lifting her to her feet. "Where's Georgio?" she inquires through her dazed confusion. "Hey, we're the ones who saved you!" shouts the boy. "You saved me," rejoins Cabiria ungratefully. "Now I wanna go home!" And that is exactly what she does.

Headstrong, no doubt, Cabiria is nonetheless operating under co-opted powers and yardsticks: her life is not yet her own.[10] Once returned to her tiny but prized home "past the gas company" (proof of Cabiria's physical existence, measure of terrestrial success) on the outskirts of town, she is too ashamed to confess to her friend Wanda what has occurred. Drenching in embarrassment and water and indignity, she claims, quite absurdly, to have fallen into the river by accident and says preemptively, "If you see Georgio, tell him I'm here." Wanda is too smart for such dissemblance, however, and quickly surmises the truth. She too is a prostitute, after all, and well-inured to street life with its attendant violence and tactic and greed. It is not until Wanda sets out for work later that evening that Cabiria cries out after her in humiliation: "Someone would throw you in the river for forty thousand lire? Drown you for forty thousand lire?" "Nowadays they'll do it for five thousand," Wanda responds curtly. "Someone who loves you?" opines Cabiria. But Wanda is no sentimentalist when it comes to matters of romance and the interchange of fluids and funds between predators and prostitutes. "What love?" she counters. "You met him a month ago. You don't know his name or where he lives! *Can't you understand? He pushed you in*!" A well-trained reality therapist if ever there was one, brief psychotherapy in all its inglorious action.

Cabiria's baptism, then, is clearly subliminal. She cannot yet envision the prospect of change and wants only to be reconciled with a man who has just tried to kill her for cash. Still, we hear the faint murmurings of possibility when, sitting alone on her front steps following Wanda's departure, Cabiria pauses just long enough to allow the emergence of suppressed awareness and dread, preludes to movement and change. She utters the words meditatively as if they have perhaps issued from some other region and sphere: *"What if I died?"* What if I died? Is it not the question which is forever rattling amid the back burners of consciousness, the superego's more pointed admonishment to the paltry lives we too often lead, early utterance of the budding apprehension of death and rebirth symbolism in which we shall here be immersed and reworking?[11]

In an instant (and for the time being it is *only* this instant) Cabiria's entire mode of being and consciousness is changed as she proceeds to remove Georgio's pictures[12] and belongings and burn his clothes in a fit of pique and fury. "Never again! *Never!*" she shouts as if her personal misfortune implied the weight and wounds of wars and holocausts, something which, from the psychological point of view, it surely does. "Who's gonna feed you now? St. Peter? Eternal love! You dirty *vitelloni!*"[13] Existential awareness as a prod to indignation as a prod, in its turn, to the principles of furtherance and resolve and pursuance.[14] And so Cabiria is through with one more man but there is as yet no substantive or lasting change, merely what Kierkegaard had called the "rotation method," a karma-like rolling of the endless wheel of destiny and role-playing and musical chairs. Later that night, our reluctant initiate is back on the streets of the *Passeggiata.*

Death and rebirth as yet almost wholly unconscious, Cabiria is at once taken up along with the others with how the prostitute Marisa, under the capable management of the pimp Amieto, has been able to procure a Fiat with proceeds from the sale of favors and drugs. Cabiria waxes rhapsodic about "imagology"[15] and the fascination with material goods, commercial replacements for an atrophied interior and more genuinely intimate life which have come to dominate the modern and mental landscape and domain: *"Of course, a Fiat is quite the thing. People think you're somebody–maybe a secretary or a daddy's girl. Watch how the men chase after you!"* Notice how the car changes nothing in the protagonist's consciousness and vision. Possessions are but a means of enhancement of reputation which, in turn, increase one's collateral in the marketplace of everyday relations and design.

There is for the moment only one voice that stands apart, that of the aging, raving Matilda–a parody of the prostitutes but more nearly some amalgam of street person and seeress who mocks the prostitutes from afar. *"Notice the difference between you and me!"* she shouts at the women. *"Look how you'll end up, you lousy whore!"* she yells, feigning now the gestures of a beggar. It is clear that the madwoman is directing her taunts specifically at Cabiria as she continues to pantomime the panhandler and hag: *"Please, for my Georgio's sake!"* Like any lunatic worth her salt, there is something of the clairvoyant in Matilde and Cabiria cannot easily broach such prophecy. With the mention of Georgio's name, she is unable to contain herself and lunges at the messenger because of a message which rings unnervingly true. The two women engage in combat (still more entertainment for the men in attendance) until the fight is finally broken up by Wanda and the others and Cabiria is driven off in Marisa's brand-new Fiat, the pimp Amieto comfortably at the wheel and in charge.

Amieto, of course, tries to enlist Cabiria under his aegis. (*"You're not doing it right. Who's watching over you? Why not find yourself a serious man, respectable like me?"*) But Cabiria seems finally to have had it with self-serving men and rather demands to be dropped off at the upscale Via Veneto,[16] where she tries, in Masina's irrepressibly comedic manner, her hand at working the more chic part of town. It is here that she meets the movie star Alberto Lazzari, suave but jaded, who picks her up after a fight with his stylish girlfriend outside a posh nightclub. Biblical overtones are deliberate and unmistakable with Lazzari clearly intended as a resurrective figure. Frank Burke (1996, p. 87) elaborates:

> (Lazzari's) occupation enables him to move from one character and movie to the next. He is not only resurrective, he is resurrectable. In the course of his appearance, he is virtually brought back to life by Cabiria (the first time she significantly affects her world), as her company dissolves his surly self-centeredness and makes possible his reconciliation with his girlfriend, Jessy. With the appearance of Lazzari, death and resurrection evolve beyond mere physical events that Cabiria passively experiences. They become something that can be envisioned, made to happen.

This is all quite true and observant. Cabiria has fallen under the spell of the handsome actor, though not so much that she is not able to perceive even here the threat of male domination and sanction as Lazzari begins by barking two-syllable orders at a woman whose name he has not even bothered to learn. *"What's all this?"* she demurs. *"Get out, get in, get in, get out! Not for me!"* But the allure of illusion afforded by a movie star whom she imagines to be "wonderful" is simply too much to resist.[17] Cabiria is temporarily lost in Lazzari's aura and fiction and remains by his side as they drink and dance into the night.

Lazzari's home is a mansion, his bedroom an actor's world of closets overstuffed with fine clothes and mirrors everywhere–the accouterments of the societal icon, a man with an audience but without substance or passion. It is only when he listens to Beethoven's very spiritual Fifth (*"I'm crazy about it,"* he confesses) that Lazzari is elevated beyond image and the commonplace and resides momentarily rapt before beauty and the divine.[18] But Burke is right: Cabiria has–like Oedipus transformed at Colonus–the power to bestow grace upon those she encounters even as she herself remains without notable solace, her struggle existing on essentially different and higher ground than that of her interlocutors. And so, when Jessy comes knocking predictably at Lazzari's door, Cabiria is whisked off surreptitiously to the bathroom (itself an ornate appendage of the visible world which rivals Cabiria's own house in sheer size and outclasses it obscenely in overdone opulence) still yielding to a world of men and now women but most of all further posturing and pretense and the playing of roles. Through the camera lens of the keyhole,[19] Cabiria watches wistfully as the famous actor and the glamorous girlfriend reconcile, however superficially, with timeworn lines they both know now by thoroughly enervated hearts. What is real if the actor always acts?

And it is further true that Cabiria herself has lived a life premised on the playing of parts for others (what else *is* prostitution and how many men or women do you know who at some level do not succumb to its ethos and influence?)[20] and so waits deferentially for the reunited lovers to play out their scripts before making her escape from the makeshift screening room of a movie star's lavatory. She has fallen asleep (another baptism and "going under" catalyzed by yet another glimpse into the futility and, indeed, horror of everyday relations) but awakens now to stare through the window into the distance and dawn of budding consciousness and light[21] rather than back to the physical room and realms with their world-weary inhabitants and false embrace, this-worldly phenomenon with which our heroine is only too well acquainted. Cabiria searches now for bona fide enlightenment and self-overcoming, matters, in the end, that are deeply personal and not merely the mechanical reproduction (a phonographic recording) of another one's (Beethoven's) bliss.[22] Burke (ibid., p. 89) here too puts it well: "For the first time, [Cabiria] looks *beyond* rather than at her world."

To be sure, such newfound perspective is never easy for one who–again, like the rest of us–is accustomed to seeing only a few inches in front of the proverbial nose, and Cabiria proceeds to bang her head harshly on a glass door on her way out of a ponderously labyrinthine mansion that might have come out of the pages of Kafka or the New Testament (*father's house has many mansions*) in its outlandish endlessness. Cabiria's perspective has at least changed, if not her vision! *"How do I get out of here?"* she mutters to herself. Is it not the question of naiveté and hope that every seeker must eventually ask: Kafka[23] and Cabiria, the director himself, the poetess laureate[24] and, God knows, we ourselves too? We read in Jung (CW 8):

> But we cannot live the afternoon of life according to the programme of life's morning; for what was great in the morning will be little at evening, and what in the morning was true will at evening have become a lie.

And we take note that it is her head that Cabiria bangs rather than some other part of the body: the awakening of consciousness or, as Buddhism would have it, "mindfulness."[25] Cabiria is moving forward and upward. We can expect some pain.

Back at the *Passeggiata* the following night, our heroine is clearly ambivalent about her incipient awareness.[26] When the other women talk casually of attending a pilgrimage to *Madonna del Divino Amore* (a shrine dedicated to the Holy Madonna and thereby symbolic of divine love and grace and the feminine which is central to Cabiria's struggle and quest), we sense the insignificance of the unthinking religious gesture and cliche: it is ritual and distraction for the group, mere entertainment. "Let's have some fun, Cabiria," exhorts Wanda as she tries to enlist her friend's participation. (Observe that it is not *merely* men who are the problem but rather *inauthenticity* and *fear of movement*, a psychological stalemate that cuts beneath blithe distinctions of gender and political expedience.) We do not blame her, however, if Cabiria is not much interested in fun. It has been barely a day since a man tried to kill her for forty thousand lire and subsequent adventures have been urging a change. Having temporarily abandoned romance as elixir, Cabiria cannot *consciously* imagine for what she would pray. "I'll think about it," she says in all artlessness and innocence. "But what would I ask for? Haven't I got everything I need? I'll even be done with the mortgage soon. I might go anyway. I haven't said no." This is perfect! It is the ambivalence in the face of change we all know first-hand and which is part and parcel of every psychotherapeutic endeavor.[27] Note, too, the misguided conflation of the mundane and ontological realms and the occlusion of the spiritual. It was Freud, states Rank (1930/1998, p. 3), who "shut out the soul."[28]

And yet Cabiria, to give her due, is truly on the cusp of change. She has found, as Karen Horney (1942) puts it, "incentive to grow" and approaches, like a client opening up to the dangers which inhere in trust and therapy, the moment of readiness for change with proper humility before uncertainty and future: Jung's "feeling toned complex," Kierkegaard's "leap of faith." And so, whereas her friends initiate the idea of attending the pilgrimage to the shrine, one senses that such holy journeying means something distinctly different for Cabiria than for the others. This will be no token homage (neither rote obeisance to institutional authority nor ecclesiastic interlude or frivolity) but more nearly the thing in itself: a quest for truth and self undertaken with a faith and will which, at these heights, is the prerogative typically of individuals rather than conglomerates. As a small procession of supplicants bound for the holy event suddenly passes by night birds busy with the nuts and bolts of making a living, Cabiria is transfixed. Her gaze is cast once again in more nearly the right direction, at the possibility of divine- and self-love rather than back to the disheartening prospects for sameness and role-playing and continued contrivance. Cabiria is in search of something else now and knows it; consciousness is now "fringed by a more" (James,

1914). As the pilgrims pass from view, Cabiria's eyes follow, her thoughts filled, one senses, with longing and sadness and possibility. There is but one kind of love, taught St. Theresa of Avila: Seek and you shall find.[29]

As Cabiria is lost in reverie, a man drives up behind her in a truck, its cargo space protected from the rain and the elements with drab sheets of canvas. Fellini is here quoting from his earlier film, *La Strada*, in which Gelsomina[30] allows her life to be defined utterly by the strongman Zampano as he sweeps her away on his American-made motorcycle with its almost identical appendage. The rain, the mud, the dismal street with its dissipated daily round, the timeworn pilgrimage of institutional adherents, the gruff-speaking truck driver who offers a lift: all appropriate intimations of Gelsomina and Zampano and the flattened rhythm of the everyday trail, a relative low point in Cabiria's dark night of the soul. And yet the story has grown more subtle and hopeful even as the director himself has struggled and grown. Cabiria is learning what can be had from men at the wheels of pickup trucks and motorcycles, too full of themselves, what can be had and what cannot. She is, at last, "within hearing distance," as we borrow here from Robert Coles (1999, p. 23), and about to take a journey Gelsomina never knew.

The newly-restored seven-minute sequence known as "the man with the sack" which follows turns a profound psychological study into an aesthetic, moral, and even spiritual gem. We see Cabiria walking through the not-yet-dawn on the outskirts of Rome looking for a "short-cut" about which the truck driver has apparently informed her. The more skeptical among us are already made uneasy by this talk of metaphorical expedience through such difficult terrain as we hear now only Cabiria's internal monologue. (*"I've been walking for an hour. Who knows where I am!"*) Suddenly the headlights of a car are seen coming toward her. A man gets out with a large sack and approaches ominously through the dark. Cabiria steps back in alarm as the expressionless man too pauses briefly and speaks to her (*"You live in the caves too? I've never seen you before"*) before continuing laconically on his way.

Cabiria does an about-face and begins to follow this strange and taciturn man who could take or do anything he desired under the circumstances but seems for a change to want nothing at all. She tags along as the man with the sack proceeds to distribute blankets and food in the early morning to the broken and dispossessed souls living in caves and craters outside the city, far from the glitter of Via Veneto and the self-absorbed patter of the streets. The man knows these homeless people by name (something the movie star couldn't quite manage)[31] and his exchanges with them are genuine and terse and unaffected. Cabiria looks on in utter amazement. (*"Who is that guy? But who is he? With some charity?"*) And, indeed, the irony is not lost upon us that the film's sole portrayal of true love has for the moment nothing to do with romance or sex or even theology but rather issues from something far more rare and important and what wise women and men and sages of all times have simply called "care."

Cabiria stops short when she sees a woman step out of her crevice to meet this unaffiliated saint who seems to be an emissary from another time and place, one who retains only so much affiliation with the earth and its suffering as to feel a sort of transpersonal[32] attachment and who comports himself with Buddha-like simplicity and grace. Cabiria is overwrought when she recognizes the decrepit old woman whose sole interpersonal life now revolves around this quiet man's thrice monthly visits and offering of alms. *"Bomba!"* she exclaims. *"Bomba! But I knew this one! Bomba, you live here?"* To be sure, Bomba is one of Cabiria's own, a former prostitute who once had charms and looks and possessions in abundance but is now reduced to inhuman indignity and squalor and the body's unrepentant decline. Bomba runs her hands through her unkempt hair with odd affectation as she recalls her former grandeur in sympathy with Cabiria's presence and memories. "I wish I had everything I used to. A place in Rome, a place in Ostia. Showered with gifts, money in the bank, jewels and gold!" "She's not lying, you know," confides Cabiria to the man with the sack. "Who'd believe it now, but this one in her day–" As we watch, we recall Matilde's prophecy (*"Look how you'll end up, you lousy whore!"*) and are wise to think not only of Cabiria but also ourselves.

When the man with the sack has completed his ministrations he gives Cabiria a ride back to the city with its attendant noise and restlessness, its own kind of squalor. The conversation is hesitant yet meaningful as Cabiria remarks on all that this man does for the poor. The man replies with reticence and selflessness: "Not as much as needed." She asks how he came to do what he does (*"But how'd you get the idea?"*) for such action and service are so many light years removed from her daily experience and, indeed, most of ours. *"I don't know myself,"* responds the man with the sack. *"Like that. Little by little."* In other words, slowly and honestly and without shortcuts or distractions or political/theological abstractions which are more typically the norm.[33] "Are you alone?" inquires the man with the sack. "My father and mother died when I was little," Cabiria answers. "I came to Rome later." "Go now and get some sleep," says the unaffiliated saint as he drops her off in the tumult of downtown Rome and quietly goes his way.[34]

And thus ends the hallowed seven-minute sequence of the man with the sack which contains the hidden message of Fellini and Jesus and Mary and, indeed, all the world's wisdom teachers–the inexorability of suffering and time and bodily decline and ultimate death but also the redemptive and biblical "still, small voice," the prompting of a spiritual sort of attunement and love and the responsibility for the other and stranger which follows, assuredly, as a matter of course. In Stephen Mitchell's (1989) appropriately egalitarian translation of the first psalm we read:

> Blessed are the man and the woman
> who have grown beyond their greed
> and have put an end to their hatred
> and no longer nourish illusions.
> But they delight in the way things are
> and keep their hearts open, day and night.
> They are like trees planted near flowing rivers,
> which bear fruit when they are ready.
> Their leaves will not fall or wither,
> Everything they do will succeed.

And there is, too, the Carmelite, St. Theresa:

> This love is always active and looking for what it can do. It cannot remain shut up in itself. Just as water, so it would seem, cannot stay locked within the earth but must seek its outlet.

Or, if you prefer, the cabalist's parlance (for, really, any translation will do):

> *Tikkun*: to heal, repair and transform the world. All the rest is commentary.

Cabiria has finally met someone who is really "wonderful" and who is no actor and it was not on Via Veneto or even in a famous man's lavatory and whom she will not see again and yet has pointed out a way: spiritual encounter even outside the Church.[35]

The meeting with the man with the sack serves as another station of the cross in Cabiria's movement toward discernment. By the time of the procession the next day she is still more aware, more committed than ever to the possibility of ascendance and advance. At the scene of the shrine, she tells Wanda that she is "going to ask the Madonna for mercy too–like you said." But whatever Wanda may have told Cabiria in confidence is now lost in the chaos of the mass and absorption of the moment as she responds dismissively that she plans to ask "for a villa in Peripli." Wanda wants only a fancy pad in the right part of town, not much better than a handsome actor or Fiat, really! "That wasn't what you wanted to ask for," Cabiria reminds her. "Don't you remember?" "I'll ask for what I want," is Wanda's curt reply. "I can change my mind, can't I?" ("*Spiritual imagination*," understates Harold Bloom, "*is hardly a universal endowment*.") And, to be sure, the votive crowd is teeming with desperate and desolate faces (they are mostly women's) all imploring something for which the outcome is by no means guaranteed.[36]

Fellini's camera eye focuses on one supplicant in particular. It is a cripple, Amieto's uncle, another man who has spent his life and made his money in the sale of women and drugs. Worn down by time and profligacy, this man hopes against hope to be restored to health and at least physical vigor and attempts now to leave nothing to chance as he proceeds to calculate like a psychologist: "Thirty masses at one thousand lire each–that's thirty thousand." That plus the solicitous purchase of candles for himself and the others makes the sum even higher. "I gave thirty-five thousand lire!" he proclaims as if to entreat that higher altitudes take note. Amieto, who has learned well the value of money and token gestures of kindness, replies in similarly pedestrian manner: "That was a good idea, uncle." (*"Ah the old questions, the old answers,"* says a character out of Beckett. *"There's nothing like them."*) Neither uncle nor nephew (*"look how you'll end up"*) has understood that transcendence is ultimately a matter of acceptance and smallness and letting go, that heaven is not taken by force.[37] The tension mounts (*"Amieto, will the Madonna bestow. Her grace on me?"*) as the old man relinquishes his crutches at the anointed moment and collapses to the ground. We are not shocked, Fellini's church is not Lourdes.

Jung (CW 10) comments insightfully on theological confusion and irony:

> Curiously enough, the Churches too want to avail themselves of mass action in order to cast out the devil with Beelzebub–the very Churches whose care is the salvation of the *individual* soul. They do not appear to have heard of the elementary axiom of mass psychology that the individual becomes morally and spiritually inferior in the mass, and for this reason they do not bother themselves overmuch with their real task of helping the individual to achieve a *metanoia*, a rebirth of the spirit.[38]

Rebirth of spirit is, to be sure, what is at stake and what makes Cabiria's struggle and quest of a piece with innumerable and often nameless itinerants who have gone before and will come again. And Jung is right to stress the solitary angle: relations are changed as one advances upon the psychospiritual incline and premature liaison may well forestall progress. Cabiria's way, like the mystic's, is often the way of loneliness and hardship and individual effort. By clinging to gratuitous orthodoxies and methods (what Fromm-Reichmann, speaking of shibboleths and standards closer to home, had aptly called "professional pompousness") the cripple effectively forfeits opportunity.

Cabiria's own moment of prayer is more private and genuine, though no less poignant or searching. She solemnly approaches the image of the Madonna (there are, for the moment, no male deities in sight) and prostrates herself. *"Change my life!"* she cries out, kissing the ground before the holy icon. *"Grant my prayer, too. Help me change my life!"* It is a heartrending display of depletion and yearning for which antidepressants will surely not be enough–a striving, as we are here too guided by Coles (1999), "toward the sacred."

Following the processional, Cabiria is with Wanda and the others on grounds adjacent to the shrine as they eat, drink, joke and otherwise enjoy a post-liturgical picnic.[39] Only Cabiria remains aloof. "I'm thinking," she responds when the rest try to draw her back to their raucous festivities. Amieto taunts her: "Don't think so hard. You'll split your head!"[40] But Cabiria has already sensed the rift between everydayness and imminence[41] and laments: *"We haven't changed! None of us has changed, Wanda. We're all just the way we were before, just like the cripple!"* In the distance she sees the small band of pilgrims returning from the shrine, marching still faithfully beneath their tattered banner and shroud. Cabiria intuits at once the insufficiency of the prescribed ritual and pilgrimage and mocks them now just as Amieto has mocked her: *"Look at those little nuns! Where are you going with that banner? Looking for snails? Did the Madonna grant you mercy? Did she?"* Note, here again, that both women and men discourage Cabiria from her quest, something which strikes us as truer to life than neat designations of sensitivity and callousness, goodness and evil, beneficence and restraint: individuation is always the exception and, as such, beyond category and groupings and pro forma reductions. "You're blind drunk," her friends say to her, the idea that the failure of prayer might be cause for anything more than fleeting inconvenience or letdown quite foreign to their own sensibilities and experience. "Drunk, ha!" Cabiria responds. "If you only knew!"[42]

Cabiria has made another step forward. When we see her next she is not back on the *Passeggiata* but rather standing alone in front of a bleak entertainment theater called The Lux, its very name emblazoned in electric lights above a dreary facade identifying it as a burlesque of, and rehearsal for, a more genuine sort of transition and light. Inside it is all show business but show business with a twist. On stage an elderly entertainer[43] runs through his magician's routine, cheap imitations of death, rebirth, and renewal. He calls now for volunteers for his scientific investigations into "magnetism, hypnotism, and auto-suggestion" as several men in the audience eagerly oblige. The entertainer asks also for a woman's assistance (*"We now need a representative of the fair sex–perhaps you, signorina?"*) and proceeds to cajole Cabiria's cooperation as hecklers from the crowd add to her hesitation and discomfiture. "They're all tricks!" Cabiria rejoins as she goes up to the stage nonetheless.

For his first "experiment," the hypnotist sets up a sailing scene on a boat which he christens the *Intrepid* with the male volunteers at the oars. The magician's powers are considerable as he orchestrates the fantasy and trance.

(*"The sea is calm and transparent, the boat is ready, and the weather is fine."*) But suddenly comes the storm (*"It's the open sea now, the waves are swelling, hear the wind whistle!"*) and, at once, it's "every man for himself" as the crew now disperses into chaos, genuflection, and fear. Even Cabiria, who looks on from the side of the stage in disbelief, is impressed at the spectacle. There is no evidence, however, that she or anyone else apprehends the deeper symbolism which the conjurer Fellini has implied: that the *Intrepid* represents a naïve faith in the shared world of the daily round (the child's belief in the certainty of one's gods and calm seas and clear sailing) and the storm the inevitability of shipwreck that each of us must necessarily suffer at points along the way. The fantasy thereby points us, yet again, in its depiction of movement and breakdown and incompleteness, toward self-overcoming and the light of awareness and what James had called "the void beyond."

Cabiria is about to follow the men back to their seats when the conjurer stops her. He has not completed his performance and has still further tricks up his sleeve, ones more in keeping with the feminine and soular[44] aspect of things.[45] The conjurer asks a few questions about demographic concerns, ascertains that his reluctant recruit is unmarried, and removes his top hat to reveal an ominous satan's mask with its attendant horns. "Enjoying this?" he inquires mischievously.[46] The conjurer contrives now a thoroughly conventional fantasy as he introduces Cabiria (who, under the spell of hypnosis, now calls herself by her Christian name, Maria,[47] in sympathy with her unadulterated and spiritual aspects) to an imaginary suitor named Oscar. (*"The garden is quiet, lovely and in bloom."*) Cabiria is, of course, no stranger to the idea of finding happiness through the romantic alliance (indeed, it is the myth that has informed her earthly career) and she goes along freely with the fantasy and narrative. Unlike the men who have proceeded her, however, she engages it more creatively, elaborating freely as she bends to the floor to pick imaginary flowers for her new love.

The conjurer looks on, well-pleased with the performance and with Cabiria's willingness to let herself go so unreservedly, as he offers commentary: *"Picking flowers denotes a gentle soul."* He sets up a mock waltz as Cabiria proceeds to dance with her fantasized soul image while he looks on and reflects:

> The orchestra will play a beautiful waltz. I'm wealthy but I'm alone and unhappy. What good are fancy cars, long journeys and luxury hotels? Smoke and illusion!

The dance is a theme which recurs throughout the film (with this one by far the most evocative and tender as Cabiria prefers typically the rumba and mambo)[48] and which returns in all of Fellini's work. It is the *dance* now of Shiva, literally the dance of the gods connoting the fleeting step of life and rhythm of the spheres, and no one dances quite like Masina![49] Cabiria is by now thoroughly absorbed in her inner dreams and deeper self. *"Then it's true?"* she asks softy in her trance-induced rapture. *"You really love me? You're not trying to deceive me? Do you mean it?"*[50]

The whole thing is so moving, so patently sincere, so much at odds with the vaudevillian atmosphere which permeates the Lux that even the hypnotist is startled into realizing that things have gone a little too far. Cabiria had been right in saying that his was the realm of tricks, that of the tawdry and apparent, while Cabiria's fantasy springs more nearly from the depths of the self and its longing: her fugue is far beyond artifice. The conjurer (who, indeed, had fallen into a little trance of his own) now abruptly ends the charade as Cabiria, like the cripple, now falls to the floor. She awakens, like any good dissociative, without recall. (*"What's been going on?"*) But Cabiria has changed since her initial going-under along the banks of the Tiber. She gets back on her feet quickly this time almost before the conjurer is able to extend a helping hand and, hence, without so much need of commonplace (and, we may say, metaphorically masculine) solicitude and patronage.

Later that evening Cabiria is reluctant to leave the theater for fear of hecklers. When she finally does she is immediately approached by a mild-mannered and soft-spoken man[51] who has seen the performance and confides his feeling and admiration for the woman, for her innocence and guilelessness:

> Men can pretend to be cynical and persuade others that we are. Yet when we are suddenly faced with purity and candor the mask of cynicism falls way. All that is best in us is awakened.

The man speaks of his own emotional response in the face of "such modesty, such sensitivity":

> Some things cannot be touched by human vulgarity. Luckily among the stupid, jeering crowd, there is always someone who understands, who appreciates. What struck me most strongly was the fact that inside of you you kept the innocence of an eighteen year old girl.

He speaks, as the skeptical and street-wise prostitute wryly notes, as though he has "swallowed a book!"[52] Cabiria herself has earned no advanced degrees and yet knows the score. She is not one to mince words.

Most shocking of all, the man now tells Cabiria that his name too is Oscar! He politely, though persistently, asks to see her again. Cabiria (who identifies herself as "a salesgirl") demurs at first, saying that she must work and hasn't time for dalliance. But she keeps her date with this seeming knight[53] and gradually becomes entranced with a man who (much more we may surmise than Georgio) says all the right things[54] and, as she boasts to her girlfriends, "always pays." In short order, Cabiria is once again in seeming love and arranges to sell everything, even her cherished home, in order to marry and move to the country with the man who always pays. While all this is happening, we see precious little of Cabiria's suitor. It is perhaps the storyteller's way of letting us know that the transformation which we witness is essentially inward, external events providing merely the pretext for intrapsychic transformation which has taken on now a life of its own.

Strolling nearby her house one afternoon, Cabiria encounters a man of the cloth[55] who calls himself Brother Giovanni and who, not unlike the madwoman Matilde, seems to be an admixture of befuddlement, eccentricity, and wisdom. Although Brother Giovanni is, like the rest, perhaps too quick to equate a woman's well-being with home, hearth, and marriage and, like the conjurer, inquires mostly after Cabiria's status in regard to these demographics, there is nonetheless weight to his words. *"The important thing,"* he tells Cabiria, *"is to be in God's grace. Whoever lives in God's grace finds happiness."* Even he perhaps does not realize that the god of which he speaks, we may say with Tillich, is "the god beyond God," a deity beyond everyday practice, ritual, and belief.[56]

The parting between Cabiria and Wanda is sad and heartfelt. Cabiria packs her bag and carefully places atop the picture of her mother (an image of the incarnate Madonna which each of us holds deeply embedded within[57]) which had hung on the wall of her diminutive abode. *"Mama, just think–I'm getting married too!"* she says to herself but also to memory and the future as she takes her leave. As the bus pulls away, even the world-toughened Wanda breaks down and cries. Cabiria tries to comfort her friend: *"You'll see! A miracle will happen to you too!"* And with these words, Cabiria departs for the afterlife.

In a lakeside village far above sea level, Cabiria and Oscar finish a late afternoon lunch. In her hands, Cabiria clutches four hundred thousand lire, her life savings bolstered by the proceeds from the sale of her house and possessions. Oscar tells Cabiria to put the money away as he continues to play the gentleman and pay. They stroll now through the woods to a cliff which juts out high above the lake where Oscar has promised to show Cabiria the sunset. They arrive just as the sun is sinking into the horizon. Cabiria is overcome with (slightly premature) ecstasy and awe:

> What a strange light! It must be true that there's some justice in the world. You suffer–you go through hell–and then comes the time to be happy.

She looks down from the precipice (*"it's so far down"*) and suddenly imagines herself sailing.[58] Momentarily stunned, Oscar asks Cabiria if she knows how to swim. "Once I would have drowned," she says, "if they hadn't pulled me out. A man threw me in."

Cabiria turns to look into Oscar's eyes and in a flash it all becomes clear. Oscar, too, is an actor, the ultimate con man, inveterate representative of the fallen realms with all their self-serving deceptions and treachery.[59] *"You want to kill me, don't you?"* Cabiria cries out; *"For the money!"* Cabiria staggers backward as she drops the bundle of bills at Oscar's feet. She has lost all dignity and is far beyond fear. (*"Kill me–throw me in! I don't want to live!"*) She stumbles dangerously close to the edge and Oscar, who indeed had, like Georgio before him, intended to kill this woman for personal gain, now rushes to secure her. Even the sociopath is overcome by Cabiria's purity of emotion. (*"Can't you see that I don't want to kill you?"*) Oscar picks up the money and flees like the coward he is. Alone, Cabiria now falls to the ground and cries out in poverty and despair. As she lapses into unconsciousness one last time, her wail becomes the distinct cry of an infant. Cabiria's truer baptism has finally arrived, a penultimate "going under," her death and rebirth.

The final scenes of the film are images of healing, return, and renewal. As Cabiria regains consciousness, she retrieves a bouquet of flowers she had dropped and makes her way back through the dusky forest to a street quite different from the treadmill existence her forbear Gelsomina had known. She has undergone, in accordance with gnostic scripture, a "migration into newness" and has become, truly, a bride of the planet and life. (*"To be alive is power/Existence in itself,"* writes Dickinson.) The schism between self and world has at last been bridged, as have the rifts within, the travails of the ego and self now silent and still. (*"Awakening,"* echoes Bloom, *"is resurrection."*) As Cabiria walks, her leadenness yields gradually to lightness of foot, her grief to almost preternatural calm. Suddenly she is surrounded with various "others," youths who encircle her with dance and song (*"What we play is life,"* the poet Louis Armstrong had said)[60] and girls who seem to represent the innocence of childhood and the redemption of the prostituted realms and paradise lost.

The whole thing is quite strange and beautiful, as though male and female spirits alike have sprung from within. And perhaps they have.[61] It is the moment in which opacity fades and Cabiria sees into the deeper mystery of things, embracing the earth and its beauty anew. (*"It's music,"* says Charlie Parker in syncopation and counterpoint. *"It's playing clean and looking for the pretty notes."*)[62] A girl approaches and bids Cabiria *"buona sera,"* a tender word of welcome as Cabiria returns transfigured to the world. She is perhaps manifestation of that purest part of Cabiria with which she became first reacquainted under the conjurer's spell. It is the fairest of evenings, Cabiria's dark odyssey of soul at last reconciled. As our film ends, Cabiria (the teardrop under one eye a poignant reminder of wounds and wars and stigmata) peers for just an instant into the camera lens, that penetrating eye of Fellini's all but ineffable genius. Her face is ethereal and her smile radiant as we, the audience, are restored vicariously to awareness ourselves. (*"The kingdom,"* announces the hidden Jesus, *"is inside you and it is outside you."*) Barriers break down now in accordance with eternal verities of heaven and earth.[63] The moment will not last but has restored and will come again. It is the pulse of life and dance of divinity, a moment of breakthrough, epiphany, and release.

Working backwards, we have:

What a strange light! It must be true that there's some justice in the world. You suffer–you go through hell–and then comes the time to be happy.

The important thing is to be in God's grace. Whoever lives in God's grace finds happiness.

Men can pretend to be cynical and persuade others that they are. Yet when we are suddenly faced with purity and candor the mask of cynicism falls way. All that is best in us is awakened.

The garden is quiet, lovely and in bloom.

Long before Jesus and the two Marys, a Chinese mystic had written:

The entrance to the mysterious feminine
Is the root of all heaven and earth.
Frail, frail it is, hardly existing.
But touch it; it will never run dry.[64]

AUTHOR NOTE

For translations of excerpted dialogue I have worked from both the older and the newly restored prints of *The Nights of Cabiria*, incorporating sometimes the one, sometimes the other, and here and there an amalgam of the two. I have been concerned throughout to write my own piece with, we may hope, its own literary worth and have attempted therefore to preserve essayistic integrity. Fellini himself would have wanted as much as his films often diverged wildly from original sources and screenplays. Here, too, the filmmaker (in Keel and Strich, 1976) spoke like the philosopher he was:

We live in an age that has made a cult of methodology, that makes us weakly believe that scientific or ideological [concerns] have the edge over reality . . . [One] is suspicious of fantasy, of individuality, in other words of personality.

Work, to repeat, ought to be "a complete part of life" and not undertaken in "a detached, professional way." In other words, it needn't be uniformly academic or clinical.

> A film is a living reality. Sometimes its order must be obeyed, sometimes one must recall it to its own internal rhythm. I don't want to make a mystery of my work, but I would like to say that my system is to have no system: I go to a story to discover what it has to tell me.

It is the artist's approach which often yields the finest fruit and the exceedingly minor liberties here taken are done in this (patently more limited) spirit and vein. In no instance has the meaning of the film been altered in the slightest way. I have gone, rather, to our story and listened with the very best ears I could summon.

NOTES

1. Fellini's early masterpiece *La Strada* (1954) was in fact the object of no mean derision upon initial viewing by an unprepared audience at the Venice Film Festival. It is not always the case, but here for once there really was someone "among the stupid, jeering crowd" who "understood" and "appreciated." Charensol (in Keel and Strich, 1976) reacted with appropriate amazement and accolade and, we dare say, even awe: "We are definitely in the presence of a poet who is like no one else and in whom we should have total confidence."

2. Let us not be too conveniently distracted by the gendered language. Fellini is writing here in the fifties, indeed, about *La Strada* and the relationship there portrayed between Gelsomina and Zampano. In that study and inquiry encounter is time and again thwarted (and ultimately fails) because of the latter's bullheadedness and ignorance, an unthinking chauvinism which cannot bend or yield and does not wake up to the mystery of life and the feminine and the sanctity of human connection therein implied until already it is too late. Further, and for the record, *Between Man and Man* (1955) is the title of a lovely book by the large-hearted Martin Buber himself, and who among us would be so philistine as to equate this saintly philosopher's essential message with small-mindedness or pejoration or prejudice?

3. But compare Fellini's untutored genius with, for example, Allen Wheelis's (1999, p. 14) equally poetic wisdom and non-parochial style and discernment, an agnostic grace all its own:

> All voices claim to grasp reality, but I don't believe them. They sound synthetic, like those computer-made voices in electronic mail. The reality they present is widow-display, not what happens in the street. I seek the sound of a human voice. A voice that bears witness, attests the way things really are. This means a voice that has freed itself, usually with great suffering and effort, of the vast corruption of language and experience, of the cliches, the jargon, and the kitsch, of that sea of deceit and pretense in which we drift. When I hear it, I turn back to page one and read carefully. Such voices are rare, are usually drowned out by the din around us.

It is hard to imagine Freud or, indeed, even Jung writing quite like this, with this sort of unfiltered subjectivity or patent disclosure or this much remove from the crowd.

4. "Don't make me say it again," was the typical response of the filmmaker who, while widely read and extraordinarily cultured, preferred in the end–and for the profoundest of reasons–a "fragmentary" understanding of things: random and open-ended and free. "I find life," he had said, "much more interesting than books." Still, most worthy lives, these days especially, include books, and Fellini's was here no exception. His spirited, searching, and far-reaching essays are elaborated with frequent and non-linear references to Dostoyevsky and Beckett, Kierkegaard and Kafka, Bellow and Poe and God remembers who else.

5. A distinction about which Fellini, to his credit, could not and would not make. Rather, he (in Keel and Strich, 1976) had written: "Work, to me, is a complete part of life. I cannot do it in a detached, professional way." Do you understand?

6. In *The Varieties of Religious Experience* (1914, p. 508), James writes that the spiritual quest is the means whereby one realizes that a

> higher part is coterminous and continuous with a MORE of the same quality, which is operative in the universe outside of him, and which he can keep in working touch with, and in a fashion get on board of and save himself when all his lower being has gone to pieces in the wreck.

James's person and book–along with several others on whom and which we shall here be reliant as lodestars and touchstones–inform the central spirit of this essay with their endorsement of an approach to sublimity which abides no "single principle or essence but is rather a collective name" (p. 26). The very title of James's classic work, *The Varieties of Religious Experience*, as Gavin (1992) rightly notes, is itself instructive. *"Truth is one,"* teaches Hindu scripture. *"The sages call it by many names."*

7. *The Nights of Cabiria* and *8 1/2* (1963) and *Juliet of the Spirits* (1965) are obvious exceptions although the breakthroughs represented even here contrast starkly with our commoner ideas about "happy endings" and are rather portrayals of grace received after the most tortured (and tortuous) external and internal trials and events often of breathtaking psychological intricacy. Offhand I am hard-pressed to come up with any other triumphal endorsements of life or existence in the Fellini canon, though inevitably we are moved and ennobled by the tragicomic effort and struggle. Fellini himself is fully aware of the problem and the pervasive skepticism, something he indeed parodies in his penultimate *Intervista* (1987). The final shot in that nostalgic work is of sunlight filtering through an open door into a studio which is suddenly superceded by the theatre's artificial lighting system. At once we hear Fellini's (in Burke, 1992, p. 287) disconcertingly soft and lyrical voice (that voice Mastroianni had described as sounding "like a Chinese flute") saying:

> So, the film should end here. Indeed, it is finished. I seem to hear the voice of my old producer: "But why do you end like this, without a thread of hope, a ray of sunshine? Give me at least a little ray of sunshine," he begged me at the first screenings of my films. A ray of sunshine? I don't know, let's try.

As we hear these words (with their almost biblical evocations) the theatre lights dim and are themselves replaced by two spotlights (ambiguity and paradox, yin and yang, white clowns and august, masculine and feminine, art and reality, joy and despair) which now form a circle of light (the "ray of sunshine" which, indeed, the producer has implored) in front of a camera and cameraman. There are footsteps heard belonging to a man who clutches a clapboard. "One, two," shouts the man as he claps the board and a filmmaker of daimonic genius attempts yet again to articulate the boundaries of existence and the soul through the media of celluloid, image, character, and narrative and so consider once more whether it is all worth the proverbial candle in the end.

Fellini's final film, *The Voice of the Moon* (1990), is not available with English subtitles but takes up yet again the quest for the feminine in a world spun frightfully out of control. Here our protagonist Ivo, played by a youthful Roberto Benigni, is a psychiatric patient (a *real* lunatic) released from the institution because of changes in Italy's laws and Zeitgeist and manners of funding which parallel those which had earlier occurred here. Thus does Fellini afford himself a final opportunity to survey the human dilemma amid a postmodern landscape through the eyes and experience of one of life's marginal figures, one who has thereby both advantages and disadvantages over everyone else. Between the world-weary Gonnella and the youthful "holy fool" Ivo this conversation ensues:

> GONELLA: They train so that each one interprets his part perfectly. Did you see the doctor? Did you notice his suit? Indeed the typical suit of a doctor. To be more authentic than that is not possible. Yet it's faked, all faked.
> IVO: But your son?
> GONELLA: Ah, that is the capstone. We are in the realm of great art. No one could take it any further. The archetype of the son, the platonic ideal . . . It's all a fiction, only a representation, all faked. (ibid. p. 303)

It is Kundera's "imagology" [see endnote 15] taken to its most logical and frightening conclusion.

The Voice of the Moon ends with Ivo utterly bankrupt and alone in his efforts to find self and meaning and love and connection. The final scene occurs far from the machinations of town and the airwaves (their own brand of madness) and takes us back precisely to the spot which has opened the film–a field where Ivo stands beside a stone well and underneath a silver moon which (verbally!) mocks his failure:

> And what do you want to talk about, the voices, eh? Trips from one well to another? You're not happy? But it's a great gift, great luck, so-called Salvini. Double lucky. It makes me angry how lucky you are. You shouldn't understand. It's a disaster to understand. What would you do after? You should only listen, only hear those voices and wish they never tire of calling you. (ibid., p. 301)

The televisual moon now turns into the face of the woman Ivo had earlier pursued unrequitedly, who says impoliticly: "You almost made me forget the most important thing: *Pubblicita!*" ("*Time for a commercial!*") As the voice of the moon is gradually replaced with the sounds of frogs and crickets and nature, we hear Ivo say bemusedly: "I believe that if there were a little more silence, if everyone made a little silence, perhaps we could understand something." With this, Ivo sticks his head deep inside the well and our film fades into darkness. And that is it: the maestro's parting message to those of us fortunate or unfortunate enough to have been left behind!

8. A willful sense of purpose which, admittedly, has returned Cabiria, at least physically, to life. To everything its season: even the guru needs an ego to catch her or his bus.

9. Fellini will soon underscore such universal proclivity with a jacket depicting flamenco-inspired images of love and which Cabiria will don, quite incongruously, when she returns to her tiny house "past the gas company."

10. Let the reader and professional be forewarned: Fellini is suggesting that neither are our own. Prostitution is of interest to the filmmaker solely in its more (lower-case) catholic implications and contexts. He will gladly defer to his colleague Pasolini (who had indeed provided consultation on the film) concerning matters of anatomical and sociological detail about streetwalkers and night life and hooking in a film which is, to repeat, ultimately universal and spiritual in its calling and import and quest. Do not misunderstand: Fellini is *always* talking to and about us.

11. The veteran psychoanalyst Allen Wheelis (1999, pp. 105-6) articulates what is occurring and is at stake with an elegance of perception and refinement of language that Cabiria (who, as we shall see, has "swallowed no books") cannot put into words yet vaguely intuits:

> Consciousness leaves my body, moves out in time and space. I undergo an expanding awareness of self, of separateness, of time flowing through me, bearing me on, knowing I have a chance, the one chance all of us have, the chance of a life, knowing a time will come when nothing lies ahead and everything lies behind, and hoping I can then look back and feel it well spent. How, in the light of fixed stars, should one live?

We recognize here precisely the poetess Wislawa Szymborska's query (*"How should we live?" someone asked me in a letter*), a question which haunts Fellini and Cabiria and each of us too and which, the honest psychologist will surely admit, suggests no expedient response. Joseph Campbell (1971, p. 6) writes succinctly: "There are no problems without consciousness."

Of course, without consciousness neither can there be bona fide awareness or perspective. Here Sri Nisargadatta Maharaj (1973, p. 528) speaks with poetic assurance and mastery that even the psychoanalyst cannot best:

> Questioner: Is not eternity endless too?
> Maharaj: Time is endless, though limited, eternity is the split moment of the *now*. We miss it because the mind is ever shuttling between the past and the future. It will not stop to focus the *now*. It can be done with comparative ease, if interest is aroused.
> Questioner: What arouses interest?
> Maharaj: Earnestness, the sign of maturity.
> Questioner: And how does maturity come about?
> Maharaj: By keeping your mind clear and clean, by living your life in full awareness of every moment as it happens . . .
> Questioner: Is such concentration at all possible?
> Maharaj: Try. One step at a time is easy. Energy flows from earnestness.

12. Notice how the large picture of Georgio (prominently displayed and accorded center stage) is surrounded by miniature, doll-like, and subservient female represen-

tations to either side, thereby providing visual portrayal of Cabiria's co-opted psychology and consciousness and, further, evidence of Rank's point about the power of the filmic image to convey. A mere shot of the camera says it all.

13. Fellini is here quoting from his earlier film *I Vitelloni* (1953). "Vitelloni" translates literally to "overgrown calves" or "veals" and seemed to connote at the time provincial men in their late twenties or thirties who, states Burke (1996), "refused to grow up–remaining unemployed, at home, and reliant on their (mostly middle-class) families" (p. 36). The failure to grow up or evolve–let us call it "ontological fixation"–is the affliction which informs the overarching theme in the filmmaker's work. This malaise (a sort of psychospiritual "stuckness" or death) is one which affects both women and men, though Fellini invokes time and again the metaphorically feminine is his efforts to articulate and effect breakthrough and release and thereby more auspicious connections with self, world, and others.

14. "Life is born," Jung (CW 7) states presciently, "only of the spark of opposites."

15. The term derives from Czech novelist Milan Kundera (1990, p. 114-5), a writer whose dark, yet passionate and absurdly humorous, central European quest for meaning and encounter in a world which has seen better days has much in common with Fellini's vision and scrutiny. In his novel *Immortality*, Kundera writes of the conformity and reduced consciousness which typify an epoch of lost significance and which may be summed up neatly with the phrase "many people, few gestures":

> Imagology! Who first thought up this remarkable neologism? Paul or I? It doesn't matter. What matters is that this word finally lets us put under one roof something that goes by so many names: advertising agencies; political campaign managers; designers who devise the shape of everything from cars to gym equipment; fashion stylists; barbers; show-business stars dictating the norms of physical beauty that all branches of imagology [must] obey.

The author's lamentation leaves no doubt as to where his personal predilections and sympathies lie: "[I]magology is stronger than reality, which has anyway long ceased to be what it was for my grandmother, who lived in a Moravian village and still knew everything through her own experience." It is precisely this re-appropriation of one's "own experience" which will comprise Cabiria's pilgrimage and quest: a very different sort of romance from the usual kind. It is noteworthy to point out that Fellini's later work parallels precisely Kundera's pessimism about the near-impossibility of navigation through a postmodern terrain. "How should we live?" someone asked me in a letter.

16. Fellini will, of course, make this glittering street famous throughout the world with his next film *La Dolce Vita* (1960), in which a jaded journalist, played to eerie perfection by Marcello Mastroianni, will there haunt the night clubs in restless pursuit of adventure and distraction and the rich and famous. That film too will begin with religious metaphor and analogy when we witness Jesus' quite literal return to earth as he wafts through the sky over St. Peter's Square and downtown Rome in the form of a statue suspended by helicopter, one of a seeming infinity of images in the Fellini canon which it is quite impossible to forget.

17. She will soon tell Lazzari that he is "as good-looking as [his] house." Recall, however, that only hours before she had been taken in by a Fiat and some of us are,

sadly, in a position to recall just how quickly this particular make can disappoint and break down! But this point about Lazzari's sluggishness in even learning Cabiria's name is instructive. Fromm-Reichmann (1950, p. 7) states emphatically: "The psychotherapist must be able to listen."

18. We are reminded of Gelsomina's song in *La Strada* (1954) which draws her irretrievably out of the world with its attendant failure and pain and which she first hears played by *Il Matto* ("the Fool") on his diminutive violin as she rests her head on a rope in the entryway to a tent in the *Giraffa* Circus. The image of the giraffe with its elongated neck, the rope which effectively separates the head from the body, the ethereal song in stark contrast with an inhospitable earth: all metaphorical and visual and aural representations of the "head problems" to which we mortals are irretrievably heir. Gelsomina, who can find neither love nor effective means for self-renewal, will eventually leave the world entirely in sympathy with her song, something the man of the world Lazarri here does momentarily. Cabiria, by way of contrast and as we shall see, will discover a courage and capacity which neither Gelsomina nor Lazarri can quite manage and will effect breakthrough where others do not.

19. Fellini is, here again, patently deliberate about this image.

20. Consider, by way of contrast, this definition of authenticity (the diametrical opposite of prostitution and posturing) suggested by the late science fiction writer Philip K. Dick (in Sutin, 1995, p. 278-9), yet another uncanny seeker into the furthest reaches of galaxies and the innermost perplexities of self:

> The authentic human being is one of us who instinctively knows what he should not do, and, in addition . . . will balk at doing it . . . This, to me, is the ultimately heroic trait of ordinary people; they say *no* to the tyrant and they calmly take the consequence of this resistance. Their deeds may be small and almost always unnoticed, unmarked by history. Their names are not remembered, nor did these authentic humans expect [them] to be . . . I see their authenticity in an odd way: not in their willingness to perform great heroic deeds but in their quiet refusals. In essence, they cannot be compelled to be what they are not.

As Sri Nisargadatta (1973, p. 315) tells his interlocutor: "But you can see the unreal as unreal and discard it. It is in discarding the false that opens the way to the true." Does the psychoanalyst require proof? Be patient for soon he or even she will meet a man with a sack.

21. A gaze, we repeat, in search of a beyond and James's "MORE," toward what Robert Coles (1999) has called "that Another"–"a moral or spiritual kind of awareness" (p. 12). "The word *more* was a favorite of James's," writes William Gavin (1992, p. 30), "for it expressed his belief that we should never cease our moral striving." The Buddha also counseled wisely:

> It is proper to doubt. Do not be led by holy scriptures, or by logic or inference, or by appearances, or by the authority of religious teachers. But when you realize that something is unwholesome and bad for you, give it up. And when you realize that something is wholesome and good for you, do it.

22. Let us remain, here in these endnotes, for the moment in the East:

> Maharaj: Why be so concerned with others? In reality, the Guru's role is only to instruct and encourage; the disciple is responsible for himself . . .

Questioner: You are not answering my question: how to find the right Guru?
Maharaj: But I did answer your question. Do not look for a Guru, do not even think of one. Make your goal your Guru. After all, the Guru is but a means to an end, not the end itself . . . [I]t is what you expect of him that matters. . . . Now, what do your expect?
Questioner: By his grace I shall be made happy, powerful and peaceful.
Maharaj: What ambitions! . . .
Questioner: I do not grasp you fully. On one hand you say a Guru is needed; on the other–the Guru can only give advice but the effort is mine. Please state clearly–can one realize the self without a Guru, or is the finding of a true Guru essential?
Maharaj: More essential is the finding of a true disciple. Believe me, a true disciple is very rare, for in no time he goes beyond the need for a Guru by finding his own self. . . . There may be many messengers but the message is one: be what you are. (in Nisargadatta, 1973, pp. 428-31)

23. "I have an appetite," professes Kafka's (1995, p. 174) insect-man Gregor Samsa, "but not for these foods. How well these boarders eat [while] I'm starving to death." In the vestibule, however, Gregor "stretch[es] out his right hand very far, toward the staircase, as if some unearthly redemption were awaiting him there" (p. 135). No wonder Fellini had so long wanted to make a film based upon one of Kafka's works and indeed shows himself running through screening tests for the Czech writer's strange and meandering novel *Amerika* in his equally strange and meandering *Intervista*. It is relevant to note that a more accurate rendering of Kafka's short story "Metamorphosis" is simply "The Transformation." "Where, then," writes Kafka (1988, p. 399) reverently in his diary, "shall I be brought?" And where are the nutritionists for the likes of Kafka and Cabiria?

24. We refer here, once again, to the dark-hued and matter-of-fact poetry of the Polish poetess Wislawa Szymborska, an excerpt of which graces our frontispiece and, indeed, points us along our way toward a faith beyond authority, patriarch, and, indeed, even creed.

25. Fellini's work, to repeat, evidences nothing so clearly as a pervasive fascination with "head" problems and cases, and, once again, we are reminded that the issue is not merely sexual but rather something far more complex. Throughout his career, the director uses his camera eye to show bodies void of faces (hence, without individuality or substantial awareness) and heads detached from their bodies (the better to accentuate the source of the trouble but also a glimpse of longed-for relief). This mind-body polarity is represented, as we have noted, in extremity in the instance of Gelsomina and Zampano. I am reminded also of Fellini's little-known *Toby Dammit* (a quite fascinating exploration of acting and would-be evolution and release), a film studded with repeated separations of head and body. Further, and as we shall see, the theme is underscored with playful irony in *The Nights of Cabiria* when a stage entertainer performs cheap magician's tricks that, yet again, effectively "kill off" the head. ("*As you can see, ladies and gentlemen, my assistant's head has been completely impaled by daggers. There's no doubt that his head must be soaked in blood. You'll be amazed to see, instead, that his head has disappeared!*") Always we are

reminded that life and consciousness themselves are the problems about which the filmmaker will not let us forget.

26. Again we note Fellini's psychoanalytic acuity in intuiting the difficulty of change which–let us confess it– burdens doctor no less than patient, a back-and-forth motion which is the very hallmark of tribulation and growth. Proper therapeutic respect and receptivity, states Fromm-Reichmann (1950, p. xi), inhere only so far as one remains aware that the patient's "difficulties in living are not too different from [one's] own."

27. In *Psychology and the Soul,* Rank (1930/1998, p. 5) confounds the symmetry and schemes of the experts when he states:

> Deep down, we don't want to observe ourselves and increase self-knowledge. First of all, the search for self-knowledge is not an original part of our nature; second, it is painful; and finally, it doesn't always help but often is disturbing . . . Knowledge of others can be put to use; too often, self-knowledge proves a hindrance.

Of course, this is but half of a very complicated story. Karen Horney (1942, p. 23) expresses proper counterpoint in writing of "incentive toward liberation":

> The fostering of [the] phony self is always at the expense of the real self, the latter being treated with disdain, at best like a poor relation . . . [T]he more the phony self evaporates, the more the real self . . . emerges . . . by becoming free from internal bondages, to live as full a life as given circumstances permit. It seems to me that the wish for developing one's energies belongs among those strivings that defy further analysis.

We are, as Buber had noted, creatures of "the in-between." Both perspectives are needed, something both Horney and Rank were astute enough to perceive.

28. We may well think of Freud's dismissal of Rank–once his chosen son–as such an instance and act. If so, we must reluctantly look upon the likes of Jones and Alexander as having perpetrated Judas-like betrayals in their slander of the man and most likely out of envy, ego, and greed. With such a perspective, the excommunication of Rank from the "church" of psychoanalysis becomes a crucifixion in effect: a sacrifice perpetrated, yet again, by the father of the son with siblings in accomplice–evidence in itself of a shutting out of soul. The therapist for Rank was more mother than father, and close scrutiny of his work suggests that he anticipated much that we call now humanism, spirituality, and the feminine in our discipline and craft.

Still, lest we be too hard on the patriarch, we must remember that Freud (the man and not always the theorist) seems to have been quite proactive in his inclusion of women in the fold from an early point and generally beneficent here in his dealings. H.D.'s lovely *Tribute to Freud* (1965), dedicated to the "blameless physician," stands as an unabashed testament to Freud's essential integrity and decency. By way of contrast, Jung was one who never stopped talking, often with impressive displays of erudition, about anima and metaphysics and soul even as his personal life and actions and liaisons were sometimes less than laudable. In the end, we may conclude that neither man gets wholly beyond image and what Wheelis calls "master building" nor from the systems which perpetuate their names and so, staggering brilliance and accomplishment aside, fail perhaps to measure up along spiritual lines with the very best. But what would this "very best" look like and how would one know when it was found? Fellini will soon render a poetic portrayal of a quiet and unassuming man, one far removed from the systems of Vienna and master builders of the Vatican and who rather evidences remarkable simplicity of spirit and modesty of soul–"a coming and going," states Beckett, "in purposelessness."

It is right, if perhaps inconvenient, to further recall that it was also Jones who found in H.D.'s book "the most enchanting ornament" of all the riffs upon Freud, "surely the most delightful and precious appreciation of Freud's personality that is ever likely to be written." This does not obviate his mistreatment of Rank but is nonetheless worthy of note: few of us really *are* the man or woman with the sack and exist somewhere between rather than beyond good and evil. Fellini (in Keel and Strich, 1976) himself says as much and with typical verve:

> There is a vertical line in spirituality that goes from the beast to the angel and on which we oscillate. Every day, every minute carries the danger of losing ground.

It is an essentially inward struggle with which we are here concerned and, in keeping with the mysterious verities and vagaries of irony and paradox, only the humble and unself-conscious gain admittance and advance.

It is further instructive to recall that my own beloved Boston had too readily and easily followed Freud's "marauders" in their haughty disavowal of Rank, an example of the professional arrogance and error which a bit too often typifies the local scene. Rollo May (in Kramer, 1996), who had left the East Coast in his later years for California, said only months before his death that he had "long considered Rank to be *the* great unacknowledged genius in Freud's circle." We are indebted to lone guns like this who set records straight and urge retrospection and scrutiny, surpassing examples in themselves of what is possible. Here as elsewhere, then, proverbial (dare we say "Rankian"?) soul-searching is urged from whence proper humility and respect will surely follow.

Let us remember, too, that Rank's excommunication by the herd had (as it did for Jesus and will for Cabiria) the unintended result of furthering solitude and travail but ultimately allows for the moment of breakthrough: direct encounter with mystery and cosmos, Buber's "I and Thou." Note too that (again like the two aforementioned but no more so than for Moses and St. Theresa and Buddha) Rank returns from epiphany to the earth and its minions as he travels first to Paris and then to the States where he rambles back and forth reading Twain and sends postcards back to the motherland simply signed "Huck." He had, like his spiritual compatriots, broken significantly out of institutional confinement in humble and almost Zen-like affiliation with an ever-changing All or Beyond or the Tao. "Read my books and put them away," he once advised an admirer. "Read *Huckleberry Finn*, everything is there." The Viennese misfit had traveled no mean distance toward becoming, truly, a man with awareness and a conscience and a sack.

Let us conclude this tangent and reverie with the reminder that the hallowed seven-minute sequence known as "the man with the sack" which we will soon consider was originally cut by producers (concerned mostly about the length of the film and their profits) after initial screenings of *The Nights of Cabiria* under apparent influence of the Vatican (which knew enough to be suspicious of the iconoclasm with which the director approached holiness and awe and divinity). Fellini had said that it broke his heart to see his own films after they had been released for they had been fashioned with such care and devotion and nuance only to be manhandled by those who had put up the money and now sought a return for their troubles. It is a redemptive and, indeed, miraculous event in itself that the missing scene should be found somehow in Paris after all these years and restored to its rightful place. And it is further fitting that our film's hidden message and teaching should be heralded by such an unaffiliated soul as the man with the sack. Fellini himself seems to have felt genuine compassion for the downtrodden and disenfranchised and, indeed, confessed shortly before his own death that he had spent much of his own life as a beggar, always trying to enlist monetary support for a stunning body of work which nonetheless met with less and less of the public's approval as he aged.

29. For Jung (CW 17) personality was revealed in "definiteness, wholeness and ripeness," something to be achieved rather than merely received. Again we must note that it is an articulation of but one half of a very complicated story.

30. Played, as all the world must surely know, also by Giulietta Masina. And, speaking of quotes, it is further interesting to note that Cabiria first makes her fictional debut in the company of an earlier incarnation of her friend Wanda in Fellini's very early effort, *The White Sheik* (1952). There the two prostitutes provide cameo levity and relief as they arrive out of nowhere in the middle of the night to offer solace to the crestfallen Ivan whose bride has abandoned him for the White Sheik (a character with whom she has become obsessed after seeing his pictures in the *fotomanzi* or "photo novels" which were popular in Italy at the time). It is another special moment in the Fellini canon which is perhaps less known than it should be and which takes up, with humor and irony, the themes of love and illusion, reality and image, spirit and authority which are to inform the director's more mature vision and work and which here achieves a happy outcome only by virtue of the most absurd compromises, reductions, and repression. In a sense, then, the whole of *The Nights of Cabiria* may be considered a gnostic reverie or riff on a cameo appearance by a little-known actress in a film which is seldom seen. Is there not some great insight and Zen wisdom here?

31. It is moving to note that Marcello Mastraoinni, in the documentary (Tato, 1997) made on the set of his final film by the women with whom he had shared his last decades of life, speaks of his abiding admiration for Fellini–not only for the depth and scope of his art and genius but also for his unerring knack for remembering the name of seemingly each and every member of each and every crew. Even the ever-modest and unassuming Mastraoinni was amazed! Theirs, recalled Fellini, was a friendship based on time and affinity and "total mistrust." Truly, such relationships are rare!

32. I use this term specifically because it contrasts so pointedly with the more voguish sense of the word which implies too often a kind of flight into paradisiacal health without especial concern for the earth or limitation or the stranger. My understanding of transpersonalism may not sell books or entice postmodern crowds but has the advantage, I think, of possessing a substance and meaning which does not refuse suffering or transience and can stand the deeper test of the spiritual traditions, one which receives only so far as it gives. Here I am with Jesus and Emerson and James

and Cabiria as opposed, let us say, to Wilber or Chopra or all the innumerable rest. We find better sympathy with Buber and Coles and Horney and Dickinson, with St. Theresa's "hybrid desire to have God and keep the world too." Do not be surprised if the man with the sack does not publish or perish or pipe up at the next professional debate.

33. "All noble things are as difficult as they are rare," writes psychiatrist and philosopher Karl Jaspers (1971, p. 99). And, of course, there is H.S. Sullivan (in Fromm-Reichmann, 1950, p. xiii), esteemed mentor to Fromm-Reichmann and May, who states with concision: "One can respect others only to the extent that one respects oneself."

34. "Be passersby," says Jesus in the *Gospel of Thomas*. "Toss wisdom and holiness onto the garbage heap," writes his forbear Lao-tzu, "and everybody will be better off."

35. Dylan's (1965) *"But to live outside the law you must be honest/I know you always say that you agree"* in a song entitled, fittingly, "Absolutely Sweet Marie." Horney (1942, p. 24) too writes of an "awe of specialization" which "paralyze[s] initiative":

> We are all too inclined to believe that only a politician can understand politics, that only a mechanic can repair our car, that only a trained gardener can prune our trees . . . Faith in specialization can easily turn into blind awe and stifle any attempt at new activity.

This, of course, is the *wrong* kind of awe and the umbrella to which Cabiria clutches in scenes even when "the weather is fine" provides a metaphorical reminder of the occluded perspective and vision which results from such abdications of responsibility and freedom. Organizational umbrellas do indeed protect us from "elements" (within and without): a very mixed blessing.

36. In his early and existentially profound novel *The Late Matia Pascal*, Fellini's compatriot Luigi Pirandello (1904/1964, p. 164-5) elaborates on the beseeching theological gesture and ploy:

> Many people still go to the churches to find the proper fuel for their little lanterns. Most of them are poor old people, poor women to whom life has lied . . . [T]hey go forward in the darkness of our existence with their feelings glowing like votive lights which they carefully protect against the cold breath of the last disillusionments . . . They hurry towards it, their eyes on the flame, thinking always: *"God sees me!"* so as not to hear the din of life around them, which rings in their ears like a string of blasphemous curses. *"God sees me . . ."* Because they see him, not only in himself but in everything, even in their poverty, in their sufferings, which will be rewarded in the end.

Pirandello's preoccupations with the ambiguity of identity and the vagaries of reality and illusion presage many of Fellini's (especially later) themes despite the director's inclusion of the playwright in a list of dislikes which included "film festivals, interviews, music in restaurants, ketchup, and 'hearing people talk about Brecht over and over'" (in Bondanella, 1992, p. 26). God bless (no pun intended) those Italians and their heartfelt expression and their humor and art.

37. Must rather, as Coles (1999) observes, be "simply summoned" rather than purchased wholesale or otherwise coerced.

38. These are no doubt fine words and the profoundest of ideas but no more so than those of Fellini himself when he speaks (in Keel and Strich, 1976) of "emancipation from conventional schemes," a retrieval "of life rhythms, of life modes, of vital cadences"–the idea, he writes, "found in all my films." "When someone says that 'God is death,'" asserts the filmmaker, "it means merely that the demand for God is seen in a purer, more uncorrupted form . . . Man is not just a social being, he is divine."

39. "The social goal," teaches Jung (CW 8), "is attained only at the cost of a diminution of personality."

40. "Good cheer," teaches Coles (1999), is "a hallmark of [a] time" (p. 145) dedicated to the "spiritually indifferent, if not callous" (p. 22). He is speaking, at least in part, of our own.

41. We may also say immanence.

42. Drunkenness, of course, is a matter of reduced consciousness whereas Cabiria's, as we have said, is now "fringed with a more." In Wheelis (1999, p. 248) we read:

> When home is lost and the nightmares begin, that's when one goes in quest of meaning . . . The problem has not been there all along; it came into being only with the loss of home, and the attempt to solve it is not an effort to create something new but to recreate something old. It is a quest backward. One is trying to refashion, in a form acceptable to an intellectualizing adult, the home of one's childhood.

Nothing so "challenges our self-awareness and alertness as being at war with oneself," observes Jung (CW 6). Cabiria now finds herself in "[a] room of immense quiet and inquiry, inquiry beneath the available answers" (Wheelis, 1999). It is the age-old battle and pilgrimage: a little sympathy is urged.

43. Played charmingly by Fellini's longtime friend Aldo Silvani, yet another actor who was truly "wonderful."

44. As opposed to "solar."

45. Again, we quote Jung (CW 7):

> Woman, with her very dissimilar psychology, is and always has been a source of information about things for which a man has no eyes. She can be his inspiration; her intuitive capacity, often superior to man's, can give him timely warning, and her feeling, always directed towards the personal, can show him ways which his own less personally accented feeling would never have discovered.

46. Things are about to get more interesting with the introduction of what we may call, with Rollo May (1969, p. 163), "the daimonic." "Man's task," writes May, "by virtue of the deepening and widening of his consciousness, is to integrate the daimonic into himself." Woman's task, of course, is essentially the same.

47. We know that this is Cabiria's real name from the sequence depicting Cabiria's encounter with the man with the sack. When the man asks her her name before he deposits her in downtown Rome, Cabiria responds frankly and without dissemb-

lance: "Maria Ceccarelli." This playing with names is instructive and implies a departure from original integrity and grace which, as we have noted, is the very hallmark of a prostitution and profligacy which has become all too endemic. We must each of us strive to progress along a psychospiritual incline from fallenness/paganism (viz., "Cabiria") to the sanctified and holy (viz., "Maria"), from imperial Rome to Bethlehem or Mecca or wherever.

48. Here too we note the dexterity with which the director juxtaposes the various images of dance, deftly drawing the distinction between the quotidian and sublimity. As such, the waltz may be equated with *Shabbat* or Sabbath. It is a day of rest, observes Buber (*"utter peace between heaven and earth"*), and, hence, the hallowed ideal experienced in slowness and quietude which must inform and inspire the daily round. "Freedom," states May (1981), "is the pause between stimulus and response."

49. Giulietta Masina and Thelonious Monk (the schizoid genius to whose newly-released 1964 performances at the *It Club* and *Jazz Workshop* I have been listening while writing this essay): my personal nominations for dancers of the century and perhaps the millennium. Both utterly unique and unrepeatable with a passion of heart and soul and a freedom of spirit and expression that could only come from attunement with the forces within and about and above and beneath–dampers to professional arrogance for those of us who may have never known such abandon or joy and spend too much of our lives peering into comforting textbooks and journals and measuring ourselves against organizational yardsticks and standards oftentimes comprising a cross no weightier nor reductive than any that Cabiria herself must confront and endure. Masina and Monk: unselfconscious and untutored and absolutely original, signs and gifts from above and the nemesis of technicians and the dutifully educated and trained.

50. Throughout this amazing scene, Fellini reveals not only symbolic artistry but analytical acumen that rivals the most subtle minds and recalls Jung's insight that individuation is an essentially spiritual journey along which only the individual who "consciously assent[s] to the power of the inner voice becomes a personality" (CW 17).

51. He appears almost out of nowhere, materializes from a wall and the shadows much as "the Fool" does in *La Strada*. In Elaine Pagels's (1995, p. 40) *The Origin of Satan,* the author documents "the social history of Satan," taking pains to point out that he appears initially in the Old Testament as a prod to change and is, hence, catalytic rather than the embodiment of evil. She quotes a biblical scholar: "If the path is bad, obstruction is good."

52. This is another interesting point: For the professional and graduate student, knowledge and competence are accrued, thereby earning letters and suffixes for our reputations and egos and names. For the spiritual seeker, however, the journey is often the opposite as she or he gives up distractions and various intellectual/theological accoutrements and returns without ceremony or fanfare to essentials and the elements of self. "Since I left Rimini," Fellini says in Charlotte Chandler's lovely *I, Fellini* (1995, p. 13), "I have been trying to uneducate and free myself from the encumbering baggage with which I was weighted as a child. The intentions may have been good, but it doesn't make the baggage less heavy." Shortly before his death, Rollo May wrote me a brief note: "Tillich used to say that the important things in life are not the accomplishments but the questions. I can only second that." It is Szym-

borska's point once again (*"the most pressing questions are naïve"*), the more remarkable for having come from such accomplished women and men as these.

53. Yes, as we have noted, Fellini might as easily have called his film *The Knights of Cabiria.*

54. This for example: *"The city is vast and we have so much to say to each other."*

55. He is a lay brother, actually, his status as a peripheral figure amid orthodoxy perhaps raising him in the filmmaker's estimation.

56. "Who is to say," inquires Coles (1999), "exactly where God is to be found?" As we read in the Zohar (the cabalistic *Book of Splendor*): "There is no place void of Him." And, here, Coles is surely right to caution linguistic pause and revision: "or Her or It." We are, indeed, reminded throughout our film of gnostic and cabalist traditions in which the self is the god within and the human quest and endeavor thereby, as Jung had suggested, the means through which divinity seeks its goal.

57. "The first bearer of the soul-image," writes Jung (CW 7), "is always the mother."

58. It is noteworthy that the rarefied moment is associated with the flow of waters and spirits and, thereby, the eternal rhythms of the earth and stars and galaxies. This is in contrast with the too-frequent fixity of institutions and churches with their respective shibboleths and in-groups and icons but once again in keeping with Eastern/ gnostic/cabalistic/transcendentalist traditions. In the Diamond Sutra we read: *"A Bodhisattva should develop a mind that alights nowhere."* Heraclitus also had said it: *"All things flow."*

59. "The ego," admonishes Coles (1999) with typical gentility and eloquence and appropriate opprobrium, "with no true conviction of its ultimate virtue."

60. Armstrong is preceded here by the pre-swing poet Rumi (in Mitchell, 1989) who writes:

> All day and night, music,
> a quiet, bright
> reedsong. If it
> fades, we fade.

61. *"Be a lamp unto yourselves,"* admonishes Buddha on his deathbed. *"Be your own confidence."* "If you do not get it from yourself," echoes the Zen master and disciple, "where will you go to find it?" "When you get the message," as even Alan Watts had counseled with modern-day summary and metaphor, "you can hang up the phone." Of course, Watts was not Buddha and we should grant the last word to the more legitimate saint: *"You are all Buddhas. There is nothing you need to achieve. Just open your eyes."*

62. *"Only a singer could say it/Only a god could hear;"* writes the pre-bop Rilke in his "Sonnets to Orpheus."

63. *"True religion,"* taught Mohammed, *"is surrender."*

64. I have never been entirely comfortable with the sometimes overwrought tendency toward neatly dichotomized distinctions between the sexes and would prefer at times that we might leave matters of literal concreteness to (external) politics and the harder sciences, returning thereby to those realms of psychology (with their inward poetry, politic, and calling) which are rightfully ours. For all the efforts of feminists and theorists, our disciplines are still notably lacking in nuance and soul and bona

fide communion. Is it not possible that this more subtle understanding and accomplishment remains irremediably the province of the exceptional effort and dialogue, something potentially realizable by all but not to be expediently schematized? Any woman or man who stumbles upon this essay will gain as much by substituting the phrase "the soul" each time she or he encounters Cabiria's name. (*"Cabiria is fragile, tender and unfortunate,"* announces Fellini in the trailers to his film.) Transformation of the self was a theme which preoccupied Fellini throughout his life. He explored the complexities of the struggle, its possibilities and failures, through progressive films which often focused on the turbulent efforts of a single person to find her or his particular manner and place of being in a difficult and rapidly changing world. From *La Strada* through *The Nights of Cabiria, La Dolce Vita, 8 1/2, Juliet of the Spirits* and beyond, the filmmaker explored the issue with uncanny intuition and insight with the "eternal feminine" (the words are Goethe's) symbolizing psyche and soul and the prospects for creative self-renewal and advance. We must surely admit Fellini into the inner sanctums of psychology and analysis in the end and, as such, far beyond theory, fashion, and system.

Mirabai, by the way, was a medieval Indian mystic and saint who seems to have embodied the best of inward and outward politics of femininity and soul. Stephen Mitchell (1989, p. 160) elaborates:

> A Rajput princess, married to the crown prince of Mewar, she refused to immolate herself on her husband's funeral pyre when he died. She flouted Hindu customs in many other ways; absorbed in her devotion to Krishna, she spent all her time at the temple, singing and dancing before his image, and mingling with the male devotees. Eventually, fed up with her family's harassment, she became a wandering ascetic. Her songs, like Kabir's, are still sung by the common people throughout India.

The Chinese mystic, by the additional way, was Lao-tzu, the legendary founder of Taoism. Lao-tzu was both male librarian and supreme articulator of the feminine, the words above set down in old age reluctantly (for action was not his thing), indeed gratuitously (for neither was the truck of ego and commerce), on his way out of town into wilderness and, quite like Cabiria, beyond. "How should we live?" someone asked me in a letter.

REFERENCES

Bloom, H. *Omens of Millennium*. NY: Riverhead Books, 1996.
Bondanella, P. *The Cinema of Federico Fellini*. Princeton: Princeton University Press, 1992.
Buber, M. *Between Man and Man* (R.G. Smith, trans.). Boston: Beacon Paperbacks, 1955.
Burke, F. *Fellini's Films*. New York: Twayne Publishers, 1996.
Campbell, J. (Ed.). *The Portable Jung*. New York, Viking Press, 1971.
Chandler, C. *I, Fellini*. New York: Random House, 1995.
Coles, R. *The Secular Mind*. Princeton University Press. 1999.
Dylan, B. *Blonde on Blonde*. New York: Columbia, 1965.

Fellini, F. *La Sciecco Bianco (The White Sheik)*. Italy, 1952.

Fellini, F. *I Vitelloni*. Italy, 1953.

Fellini, F. *La Strada*. Italy, 1954.

Fellini, F. *La Notti di Cabiria (The Nights of Cabiria)*. Italy, 1956.

Fellini, F. *Jiuletta degli Spiriti (Juliet of the Spirits)*. Italy, 1965.

Fellini, F. *Intervista*. Italy, 1987.

Fellini, F. *La Voce della Luna (The Voice of the Moon)*. Italy, 1990.

Fromm-Reichmann, *Principles of Intensive Psychotherapy*. Chicago: University of Chicago Press, 1950.

Gavin, W. J. *William James and the Reinstatement of the Vague*. Philadelphia: Temple University Press, 1992.

H.D. *Tribute to Freud*. New York: New Directions, 1974.

Horney, K. *Self-Analysis*. New York: Norton & Company, 1942.

James, W. *The Varieties of Religious Experience*. New York: Longmans, Green and Co. 1914.

Jaspers, K. *Philosophy of Existence* (R.F. Grabau, trans.). Philadelphia: University of Pennsylvania Press, 1971.

Kafka, F. *Diaries* 1910-1923. New York: Schoken Books, 1988.

Kafka, F. *Metamorphosis, In the Penal Colony, & Other Stories* (J. Neugroschel, trans.). New York: Scribner Paperback, 1995.

Keel, A. and Strich, C. (Eds.). *Fellini on Fellini* (I. Quigley, trans.). New York: Dell, 1976.

Kundera, M. *Immortality* (P. Kussi, trans.). New York: Grove Weidenfeld, 1990.

May, R. *Love and Will*. New York: Norton, 1969.

May, R. *Freedom and Destiny*. New York: Norton, 1981.

Mitchell, S. *The Enlightened Heart*. New York: Harper & Row, 1989.

Mitchell, S. *The Enlightened Mind*. New York: HarperCollins, 1991.

Monk, T. *Live at the Jazz Workshop*. New York: Columbia/Legacy: 1964/1982.

Monk, T. *Live at the It Club*. New York: Columbia/Legacy: 1964/1998.

Nisargadatta, S. *I am That* (M. Frydman, trans.). Durham: Acorn Press, 1973.

Pagels, E. *The Origin of Satan*. New York: Random House, 1995.

Pirandello, L. *The Late Mattia Pascal* (W. Weaver, trans.) London: Andre Deutsch Ltd. 1964.

Rank, O. *Psychology and the Soul* (G.C. Richter and E.J. Lieberman, trans.). Baltimore: Johns Hopkins University Press, 1998.

Sukin, L. (Ed.). *The Shifting Realities of Philip K. Dick: Selected Literary and Philosophical Writings*. New York: Vintage Books, 1995.

Tato, A. *Marcello Mastroianni, I Remember, Yes I Remember*. Italy, 1997.

Wheelis, A. *The Listener*. New York: Norton, 1999.

From the Couch to *The Concert:*
Streisand as Doctor and Patient

Rob Marchesani

SUMMARY. *Barbra: The Concert* marked Barbra Streisand's return to the stage after many years of struggling with stage fright. The following article examines her performance and the role psychotherapy played in her recovery. Streisand's use of psychotherapy is revealed in her production and integrates her facility to play both patient and doctor through her numerous films. *[Article copies available for a fee from The Haworth Document Delivery Service: 1-800-342-9678. E-mail address: <getinfo@haworthpressinc. com> Website: <http://www.HaworthPress.com> © 2001 by The Haworth Press, Inc. All rights reserved.]*

KEYWORDS. Barbra Streisand, stage fright, free association, creativity, movies, songwriting, unrequited love, disappointments, comebacks

Considered as a process in which patient and analyst are engaged with each other, psychoanalysis may be seen as art in another sense: The psychoanalytic situation and process involves a reenactment, a dramatization of aspects of the patient's psychic life history, created and staged in conjunction with, and directed by, the analyst. The idea of the

---

Rob Marchesani is a psychotherapist in private practice in New York City where he teaches "The Internet and the Hyper-Self" at The New School in Greenwich Village. In 1996 he appeared in the Beth B film *Visiting Desire,* a documentary on fantasy and sexual relations which entered the Toronto and Berlin film festivals after playing at Cinema Village. He holds a Masters from The New School and is co-editor of *The Psychotherapy Patient* series.

[Haworth co-indexing entry note]: "From the Couch to *The Concert*: Streisand as Doctor and Patient." Marchesani, Rob. Co-published simultaneously in *The Psychotherapy Patient* (The Haworth Press, Inc.) Vol. 11, No. 3/4, 2001, pp. 93-97; and: *Frightful Stages: From the Primitive to the Therapeutic* (ed: Robert B. Marchesani, and E. Mark Stern) The Haworth Press, Inc., 2001, pp. 93-97. Single or multiple copies of this article are available for a fee from The Haworth Document Delivery Service [1-800-342-9678, 9:00 a.m. - 5:00 p.m. (EST). E-mail address: getinfo@haworthpressinc.com].

> *transference neurosis expresses this understanding of psychoanalysis as an emotionally experienced recapitulation of the patient's inner life history in crucial aspects of its unfolding. Seen in this light, psycho-analysis shares important features with dramatic art.*
>
> –Loewald/*Psychoanalysis as an Art and the Fantasy Character of the Psychoanalytic Situation*

While watching *Barbra: The Concert* (1994), I was struck by the role psychotherapy played in the performer's life and career. It was popular knowledge that Barbra Streisand had struggled with an intense fear of the stage, although the audience would never have known it by the way she performed at Madison Square Garden, where she was confident and assured, even loving of her memories of Marlon Brando and her own son, Jason Gould, an actor who appeared with his mother in *The Prince of Tides*.

Of seeing Brando for the first time, Streisand remarked as she reminisced through an old film, "It was truly a life-altering experience." Brando himself was at the top of *The People's Almanac*'s (1975 edition) list of "20 Celebrities Who've Been Psychoanalyzed." But when Streisand took a seat on the couch, I wondered what she was up to in Act One. Was she about to depict an analysis or would this be one more parody on the work that I was trained to conduct? Although she never uses the word "psychoanalysis" throughout any of the three vignettes that depict her in therapy, in the very first one Streisand sits on the classical couch that has stood as an icon of the uncon-scious since Freud's day. In the first vignette, Streisand begins talking anx-iously about the present-day problems of dating. The audience then hears a disembodied voice from an empty wingback chair just behind the head of the couch. And a distinctly older, male voice says, "Vhy don't you just let your mind vander?"

"Vander?" Barbra gives the voice a slight double take, mimicking his unmistakable Viennese accent.

"Vander," the voice maintains.

She pauses and then relaxes into the corner of the couch closest to the chair.

"All right," she gives in willingly, even happily, wandering back to the memory of a blind date she'd had in high school.

It's hard to miss the obvious references to psychoanalysis: the couch, the voice, and the implicit reference to free association by "letting your mind wander (Viennese style)" and not add Streisand to the list of celebrities who have courageously embraced the couch and, as courageously, let go of it to live and work as Streisand did on that closing night of her tour.

From the couch Streisand breaks into song, marking a tribute to the cre-ative potential that can be released in an individual who travels through their personal history on the couch. She sings, "Will he like me . . . will he know enough to know that there is more to me than I may always show. . . ." She ends the song and takes her seat on another therapist's couch. This time, we hear the sound of a woman's voice. And once again, Barbra is there to work on relationships, as the therapist reminds her. Her story continues to unfold with the therapist simply adding when she hesitates, "And . . ." in much the same way the Viennese voice had urged in the first vignette, "Ya, go on. . . ." The therapist's voice and chair fades as Streisand and her voice once again emerge from the couch.

Yet, a third time she finishes a song about love and ends up on a chair behind the wingback from which another disembodied therapist's voice asks her, "Have you ever been in therapy before?" Streisand responds flippantly, a mixture of mild irritation and boldness, "Have I ever been in therapy before?" and looks to the audience, which is laughing. She continues, "Now I'm really fascinated by Jung, you know the collective unconscious, the archetypal triangle: father-mother-child. It all comes down to that, doesn't it?"

"Yes, it does," the therapist says. "I would think all the different types of therapy must have been very confusing."

"Yeah, with all the transference and countertransference, sometimes I don't know whether I'm the patient or the doctor," Streisand says and then proceeds to show a series of clips from her own films in which she plays analyst and patient in alternating roles. She concludes, "I don't care if you're the patient or the doctor, relationships are difficult to have. I guess the only good thing about unrequited love is that it's been the inspiration for some of the greatest songs ever written," like the one she proceeds to sing by Gershwin.

Was she referring to the relationship between the patient and the doctor that becomes so intense that it often mimics unrequited love, maybe even is unrequited love? For in the last clip of the series, Barbra, the patient, is backing out of the therapist's office with that look of endearing infatuation that only the young Streisand can show so innocently and so revealingly as she pulls the pocket doors closed and says goodbye. Our glimpse of her past is over and we return to her older self on stage.

"One of the nice things about growing older is realizing that you can survive life's disappointments," she says. "And you also realize that you cannot look to someone else for your happiness. Of course, that screws up the songs you can sing. You know, you can't sing those dependent victim songs anymore with the same conviction. . . . But there are songs that you can sing and really mean, after many hours of therapy." And she breaks into, "On a clear day, rise and look around you and you'll see who you are."

No doubt, she had come into the best of a good analysis where love and work are united. I might wish she would have used the word psychoanalysis. But, besides the props and the many inferences, "transference and counter-transference" were words enough. It looked like analysis, it sounded like analysis and in fact, it was analysis. So, I'll place my faith in what Bettelheim and Rosenfeld called psychotherapy–*The Art of the Obvious* (1993), something that any practitioner needs to learn–to trust the seen as well as the unseen.

That Streisand both wrote and directed *Barbra: The Concert* warrants further applause for the behind-the-scenes-work of analysis, where the patient conceives herself anew and directs that self in a new way, not just with the playfulness of one's childhood restored, but with the internalized parenting of the analyst who prompts that it's okay to speak up, to sing out and to be heard.

The Concert is a celebration of the triumph of the couch. And for Streisand, that means more than "truly, the greatest vocalist around," as Marvin Hamlisch, musical director for *The Concert*, said of her. It's also her presence, which is to say, her personality. Maybe Streisand's is the story of the creative possibilities of the couch, which is to say the triumph of a personal tale, composed out of many hours of revisiting and restoring memories, dreams and one's own particular imagination. As many of the best stories on stage, in film, and on the page are told through what seem to be dramatic expressions of ordinary life, Streisand's story may present the extreme of the many fears that bring one to the couch and also keep one away from the couch with the complaint, "It takes too long." For those who still believe analysis "takes too long," consider, after seeing her performance (available on tape): Was it worth the 27 years she took to make it back to the stage? Consider too, that in those 27 years she was productive on other stages, acting and directing movies.

I happened upon a piece of writing from the Cheyne Exhibition on the occasion of their twentieth anniversary held at the National Arts Club on Gramercy Park. As part of that exhibition, Cheyne editor Jean-Francois Manier wrote *In Praise of Slowness*:

> Confronted with the risk of having only 'fast food' literature
> left to enjoy, I feel an urgency to resist the growing powers
> of the entrepreneurs of culture.
>
> The book is such an inordinate life stake that it
> requires criteria of value other than the rate of its
> turnover. I believe the irreplaceable richness of the
> book comes from the slowness, the gravity of its
> making. These very constraints guarantee the book
>   its lasting freedom.

Yes, the book needs another sort of time: a time
for the writer in front of his work, a time for the
craftsman in front of the papers, the inks, a time
for the librarian to ruminate over choices, for the
bookseller to trade, and a time for the reader to
pleasure in the text.

A time, surely, for meetings to mature, for the
unforseeable metamorphoses to be completed.
Time for the slow wondering. Time for
the urgency to love.

If such time should be taken to produce books, should not the same care
and consideration, if not more, be taken with people?

What sent Streisand to the couch? Fear of her life after being threatened in
1967 when she was politically outspoken. A perfect example of what happens to many who dare to say what they think. Whether by an authority figure
in childhood or by radical PLO warriors on the streets, the damage to the
human psyche for speaking out is evident in psychoanalysis, which has been
so aptly referred to as "the talking cure" by its first patient. It has become a
process that strives to free up the will and the voice to speak and even to sing
again–to trust that life will not be taken away when patient rises again, but
rather will be shared as it was first shared on the couch. At the end of the
concert, Streisand reveals, "I've learned a lot. I've conquered some of my
fears even . . ." giving witness that patient remains as therapist, still human
and still afraid at times, but no longer paralyzed.

REFERENCES

Bettelheim, B. and Rosenfeld, A. (1993). The art of the obvious: developing insight
for psychotherapy and everyday life. New York: Knopf.
Loewald, H. (1975). Psychoanalysis as an art and the fantasy character of the psychoanalytic situation. In Fogel, G. (Ed.), The work of Hans Loewald. New Jersey,
London: Jason Aronson Inc.

Awe and Terror in the Living
of the Resolution of the Polarity
of Insight and Expression

Edward W. L. Smith

SUMMARY. Insight and Expression, two polar emphases in psychotherapy, are approached as inflections of the competing Apollonian and Dionysian world views. Having explored this in depth, a case is made that an embodied Gestalt approach to therapy, while decidedly Dionysian in emphasis, provides a resolution of the polarity of Insight and Expression. The resolution is through an experienced Gestalt which is constituted of Awareness *and* Expression. The Dionysian emphasis, however, brings with it potential awe *and* terror. *[Article copies available for a fee from The Haworth Document Delivery Service: 1-800-342-9678. E-mail address: <getinfo@haworthpressinc.com> Website: <http://www. HaworthPress.com> © 2001 by The Haworth Press, Inc. All rights reserved.]*

KEYWORDS. Jack Nicholson, William Blake, Kierkegaard, Nietzsche, Zen, fate, evolution, Apollo, Dionysus, epiphany, communication, Insight Therapies, Action Therapies, dehumanization, self-interruptions, emotion

---

Edward W. L. Smith, PhD, ABPP, holds the rank of Professor of Psychology and is Coordinator of Clinical Training at Georgia Southern University. He is a Fellow of the Georgia Psychological Association and of the American Psychological Association through the Division of Psychotherapy and Division of Humanistic Psychology. He is widely published and has traveled extensively as an international lecturer and workshop leader.

Address correspondence to: Edward W. L. Smith, Dept. of Psychology, Box 8041, Georgia Southern University, Statesboro, GA 30460-8041.

[Haworth co-indexing entry note]: "Awe and Terror in the Living of the Resolution of the Polarity of Insight and Expression." Smith, Edward W. L. Co-published simultaneously in *The Psychotherapy Patient* (The Haworth Press, Inc.) Vol. 11, No. 3/4, 2001, pp. 99-121; and: *Frightful Stages: From the Primitive to the Therapeutic* (ed: Robert B. Marchesani, and E. Mark Stern) The Haworth Press, Inc., 2001, pp. 99-121. Single or multiple copies of this article are available for a fee from The Haworth Document Delivery Service [1-800-342-9678, 9:00 a.m. - 5:00 p.m. (EST). E-mail address: getinfo@haworthpressinc.com].

Passion without precision–chaos.

–Jack Nicholson (in *The Witches of Eastwick*)

He who desires but acts not, breeds pestilence.

–William Blake ("The Marriage of Heaven and Hell")

Not operating under the constraints of a psychotherapy patois, Jack Nicholson, with that inimitable look in his eyes, summarized the relationship between passion and precision. His proclamation can be taken as a tocsin, a warning of what may happen when passion is not guided precisely, when action fueled by passion is not given benefit of insightful guidance. The result is chaos, a word meaning, in both its Greek and Latin origins, confusion and the formlessness preceding order. In his role as the Devil in *The Witches of Eastwick*, Nicholson has no dearth of passion. Filled with passion, emotion, eros, he is ripe for action, ever ready for spontaneous expression. So, coming from this side, he is well advised to call for precision, to invoke the logos.

Another Devil, C. S. Lewis's Screwtape, writing to his devil nephew on how to prevent human salvation, advised, "Keep everything hazy in his mind now, and you will have all eternity wherein to amuse yourself by producing in him the peculiar kind of clarity which Hell affords" (Lewis, C. S., 1996, p. 23). So here we have another warning of the fate that can result from lack of insight, that clarity of mind, which is required for precision of action.

William Blake is coming from the other side. His cause is that of passion and the encouragement of action. If I read Blake correctly, he meant pestilence not just as harmful or dangerous, but in its most severe meaning of virulent or fatal. Thus comes his serious warning about passion not expressed.

Kierkegaard, too, applauds the side of passionate action. He saw all about him people professing beliefs which they did not embody and live out. With sardonic tone he wrote in his diary, "Stuff and nonsense and balderdash instead of action, that is what people want," and further, "The secret of life, if one wants to get on well, is: plenty of chit-chat about what one intends to do and how one is kept from doing it–and no action" (Kierkegaard, 1993, p. 108). Kierkegaard emphasizes the doing, the existential choice to live out into the world. "What a person can understand he must also be able to force himself to *will*. Between understanding and willing is where excuses and evasions have their being" (Kierkegaard, 1993, p. 126). Knowing, believing, understanding, those things which are the ground for precision in guiding action, are of little value if not acted upon. For, "If a person does not become what he understands, he does not really understand it" (Kierkegaard, 1993, p. 126). ". . . T[he] Highest, after all, is not to *comprehend* the Highest, but to do it"

(Kierkegaard, 1993, p. 146). In all of his discussion of "willing to action," there is the implication of underlying passion. Kierkegaard posits "the leap," as opposed to a process of slow personal evolution, as the momentum that may explain the motion of our existence. And, "the leap" assumes passion (Kierkegaard, 1993, p. 226).

In the following century, we find Paul Tillich echoing Kierkegaard in his discussion of the "existential attitude." For Tillich, "The existential attitude is one of involvement in contrast to a merely theoretical or detached attitude. 'Existentialism' in this sense can be defined as participating in a situation . . . with the whole of one's existence" (Tillich, 1962, p. 652). And participation, of course, implies and includes passionate action.

In the context set by Blake, Kierkegaard, and Tillich, in which living out one's passion is highly valued, thinking, knowing, understanding–*insight*–is of little value when detached from action. In fact, such "ratiocination" may be an avoidance of action and even of feeling. Screwtape, again, instructs us, saying, "The more often he feels without acting, the less he will be able ever to act, and, in the long run, the less he will be able to feel" (Lewis, 1996, p. 57). Put most tersely, in this context "Thinking is a symptom" (Prather, 1972, no page number).

APOLLONIAN AND DIONYSIAN WORLD VIEWS

These two emphases, one on the control and insightful guidance of passion and desire and the other on the expression of passion itself, can be related to two alternative visions which appear across cultures. These competing world views have been labeled in various ways, but their elements are consistent. The first has been related to Apollo, Greek god of light, moderation, reason, truth, order, balance, and boundaries. The second vision has been related to the Greek god of excess, fantasy, and metamorphosis, Dionysus the god of wine.

Dionysus seems the more complex figure, and the symbolism of this god more mysterious. Even his origin offers complex and intriguing symbolism. Zeus was so madly in love with the Theban princess Semele that he promised he would do anything she asked of him, swearing by the river Styx, an oath unbreakable even for the supreme god. Semele said she wanted above all to see Zeus in his full splendor as King of Heaven and Lord of the Thunderbolt. Knowing that no mortal could behold him as such and survive, but being bound by his oath, he appeared to Semele as she had asked. She perished in the glory of burning light. As she died, Zeus snatched from her their unborn child. He hid the child in his side until time for it to be born so that Hera, wife and sister to him, would not know. For it was she who in her jealousy had put the fatal wish into the heart of Semele. When Dionysus was born, Zeus entrusted his care to the nymphs of the loveliest of the earth's valleys, a valley never seen by a mortal. These nymphs are believed by some to be the stars which bring rain when near the horizon, the Hyades. "So the God of the Vine was born of fire and nursed by rain, the hard burning heat that ripens the grapes and the water that keeps the plant alive" (Hamilton, 1942, p. 55).

Dionysus, as the only god not born of two divine parents, presents even in his origin a promise of mystery, perhaps even danger. Just as he sprang from two sides, one divine and one mortal, he himself shows two sides. As God of wine, fantasy, and metamorphosis, he inspires toward freeing the soul to dream, imagine, and to transform. Think of his vines, themselves. In winter they are black and withered and appear dead, but in spring they send forth their green shoots, coming into a full verdant splendor with the summer, and with summer and autumn are heavy with grapes. The metamorphosis is striking and the symbolism powerful. In addition, the grape to grape juice to wine transformation offers an equally striking and powerful symbolization of metamorphosis.

The other side of Dionysus is shown in his being the god of wine and excess. Just as wine used in moderation can lift and inspire, used immoderately it can lead to behavior of terrible excess. In one story, Dionysus, who was on a ship, took the form of an angry lion, causing the sailors to jump overboard (and to be transformed into dolphins). In another, he drove a group of women mad, causing them to attack and dismember the child of one of them (Hamilton, 1942). (This is still a problem today, as alcohol-abusing parents may terrorize their children, sometimes resulting in the children's "jumping ship.")

The gods of Olympus tended to love order and beauty in their worship and in their temples, following the way of Apollo. But the followers of Dionysus had no temples, preferring to "worship under the open sky and the ecstasy of joy it brought in the wild beauty of the world" (Hamilton, 1942, p. 57). "Frenzied with wine . . . they rushed through woods and mountains uttering sharp cries . . . , swept away in a fierce ecstasy" (Hamilton, 1942, p. 56).

While Apollo remained for the Romans what he had been for the Greeks, Dionysus became the Roman god Bacchus and the side of excess became emphasized (Partridge, 1960). Sheldon Kopp (1971, p. 74) summarized the transition in this way. "Later, when this cult of the Mad God appeared in Rome, it became debased into celebration of orgies of debauchery, rather than simple revelry. . . . Bacchanalia. . . ." In the words of Milton (Sabin, 1940, p. 38), "Bacchus, that first from out the purple grape/Crushed the sweet poison of misused wine." There is even a theory that the word "tragedy" may have its origin in "the goat-song" which was used in the worship of Bacchus. Only later, this theory purports, did the word become associated with drama (Sabin, 1940, p. 39).

The complexity of the two-sided nature of Dionysus is subtly, yet power-fully, revealed, again, in the mythopoesis. We are told (Hamilton, 1942) that Dionysus did not forget about his mother, though he never knew her, and longed for her. Therefore, he dared the perilous journey to the netherworld in order to find her. Defying the power of Death to keep her, he won, and took her to Olympus. As mother of a god, although a mortal, herself, she was allowed to dwell among the immortals.

I offer this interpretation. Dionysian ecstasy does not necessarily require the abandonment or forgetting of our human origins (or nature), even while inspiring us to great daring and noble deed. And though mortal, we can be delivered to lofty heights. Our relationship with divine ecstasy can deliver us to a realm of divine-like existence, that is, the dwelling with the divine. Another interpretation is that it is a perilous and daring task for the male to seek out the feminine (which is part of him) from his depths. But, succeeding in this task, his feminine part becomes exalted, as if divine.

Put in terms most mundane, "Wine is bad as well as good. It cheers and warms men's hearts; it also makes them drunk" (Hamilton, 1942, p. 60). "The worship of Dionysus was centered in these two ideas so far apart–of freedom and ecstatic joy and of savage brutality. The God of Wine could give either to his worshipers" (Hamilton, 1942, p. 57). Consider this, as well. Liber, an ancient Italian deity of the vine, worshipped as a fertility god, came to be identified with Dionysus and his Roman counterpart, Bacchus (Funk and Wagnalls, 1984). It is from his name, Liber, that we derive such words as "liberty," "liberation," "liberal," and "libertine." So, again, we see free-dom, being set free, not restricted, and licentiousness (indulging desires without restraint) as stemming from the same source.

Although we do not know a lot about the Greek mystery religions, the Eleusinian, the Orphic, the Dionysian, because they did remain mysteries (Campbell, 1990), we do have the mythic material concerning Dionysus. And, importantly, we have the expression of these two competing world views often referred to and so beautifully symbolized by Apollo and Diony-sus.

Moving from the mythopoetic to the philosophical, Nietzsche placed him-self clearly and strongly on the side of the Dionysian. In *Twilight of the Idols,* he declares himself boldly, "I, the last disciple of the philosopher Dionysus–I, the teacher of the eternal recurrence" (Kaufmann, 1982, p. 563). Nietzsche saw in the Dionysian the very core of the Greek veneration of life. "For it is only in the Dionysian mysteries, in the psychology of the Dionysian state, that the *basic fact* of the Hellenic instinct finds expression–its 'will to life.' . . . Saying Yes to life even in its strangest and hardest problems, the will to life rejoicing over its own inexhaustibility even in the very sacrifice of its highest types–*that* is what I call Dionysian" (Kaufmann, 1982, p. 561-562). Somewhat earlier, in speaking of the Hellenic instinct, Nietzsche refers to "that wonderful phenomenon which bears the name of Dionysus," and goes on to say that "it is explicable only in terms of an *excess* of force" (Kaufmann, 1982, p. 560).

Thus Spoke Zarathustra, Nietzsche's most popular book, is replete with examples of what Kaufmann terms "Dionysian exhuberance" (Kaufmann, 1982, p. 107). (In fact a strong case could be made that this work is an account of a Dionysian epiphany.) As an example of his regard for passion, Zarathustra speaks the following: "And whether you came from the tribe of the choleric or of the voluptuous or of the fanatic or of the vengeful, in the end all your passions become virtues and all your devils, angels" (Kaufmann, 1982, p. 148).

Joseph Campbell (1990, p. 198) offers a noteworthy summary of the meaning of the Dionysian. "The best discussion, in my opinion, of Dionysos [sic] and Apollo is in Nietzsche's *The Birth of Tragedy,* where they are shown in relation to the whole world of the classic arts. Nietzsche writes of Dionysos [sic] as the dynamic of time that rolls through all things, destroying old forms and bringing forth new with, what he terms is, an 'indifference to the differences.' In contrast to this is the light world of Apollo and its interest in the exquisite differences of forms, which Nietzsche calls the *principium individuationis.* The power of Dionysos [sic] is to ride on the full fury of the life force. That's what he represents. So, the essential message of the rites, apparently, is that of a realization in a properly prepared way of the dynamic of inexhaustible nature which pours its energy into the field of time and with which we are to be in harmony, both in its destructive and in its productive aspects. This is experience of the life power in its full career."

Nietzsche himself, in his discourse "Toward a psychology of the artist" in *Twilight of the Idols* (Kaufmann, 1982) gives us an especially valuable perspective. "If there is to be art, if there is to be any aesthetic doing and seeing, one physiological condition is indispensable: frenzy. . . . In this state one enriches everything out of one's own fullness. . . . A man in this state transforms things until they mirror his power–until they are reflections of his perfection. This *having to* transform into perfection is–art" (p. 518). (In reading these pieces which I have strung together, and in the following ones, consider psychotherapy as one of the arts, with the therapist and the person in therapy as co-creators. Add the "art of psychotherapy" to the arts which Nietzsche explicitly addresses–painting, sculpture, poetry, music, acting, dancing.) Nietzsche proceeds to distinguish the Apollonian and Dionysian forces in art. "What is the meaning of the conceptual opposites which I have introduced into aesthetics, *Apollinian* [sic] and *Dionysian,* both conceived as kinds of frenzy? The Apollinian [sic] frenzy excites the eye above all, so that it gains the power of vision. . . . In the Dionysian state, on the other hand, the whole affective system is excited and enhanced: so that it discharges all its means of expression at once and drives forth simultaneously the power of representation, imitation, transfiguration, transformation, and every kind of mimicking and acting. The essential feature here remains the ease of metamorphosis. . . . It is impossible for the Dionysian type not to understand any suggestion; he does not overlook any sign of an affect; he possesses the instinct of understanding and guessing in the highest degree, just as he commands the art of communication in the highest degree" (p. 519-520).

Before departing Nietzsche (and keeping the art of psychotherapy still in mind), I want to call attention to one more of his insights. To wit, ". . . all becoming and growing–all that guarantees a future–involves pain" (Kaufmann, 1982, p. 562). Let us not lose sight of this point in its brevity. *Nota bene*: *all becoming and growing involves pain*.

In her discussion of the Apollonian and Dionysian, within the context of psychotherapy, Karen Horney (Shostrom, 1967) identified the former with mastery and molding, the latter with surrender and drift. To her way of thinking, neither is better or worse, per se. They are two natural human tendencies. No one is completely one or the other, but rather we all lean more toward one or the other, sometimes preferring one, sometimes the other at different times. When manifesting the Apollonian leaning, the person will emphasize being in charge and in control, making things happen as he or she wants, trying to change the environment to suit his or her will. In contrast, the Dionysian leaning becomes manifest in an acceptance and surrender to what is and a "will-ingness" to be taken away, carried away, to flow with the river that is life. That river may be halcyon or it may be tempestuous, but most often arousing of passion.

At this point we can segue into the thinking of Carl Jung (1970) by mention of his discussion of the principles of "logos" and "eros." The "logos" principle is one of objective interest, putting aside emotional and personal subjective considerations. "Logos," being found both in Greek and Latin, meant the word by which the inward thought is expressed, or the thought itself. It refers to the doctrine of reason or thought as the controlling principle of the universe. Hence, "logic" and "logistic." "Eros," in contrast, comes from the name of the Greek god of love, Cupid for the Romans. Hence, "erotic," pertaining to or prompted by sexual desires, and "cupidity." Therefore the eros principle is one of affective-cum-psychic relatedness, a subjectively emotional mode of experiencing the world. Jung noted that in the Western view, this mode of psychic relatedness is usually seen as "feminine," whereas the logos principle is more often identified with the "masculine" orientation. With origin in the collective unconscious, these archetypes evolved into the psychic structures of anima (the "feminine" within the man) and animus (the "masculine" within the woman). Before leaving Jung's contribution to our understanding of the two world views, I want to offer a summary: The logos principle represents reason and objective interest, it is archetypally "masculine," its structural representation in the psyche of woman is the animus, and the ectopsychic function most related to it is Thinking. The eros principle represents psychic, affectively based relatedness, it is archetypally "feminine," its structural representation in the psyche of man is the anima, and the ectopsychic function most related to it is Feeling. The logos principle is Apollonian. The eros principle is Dionysian.

Writing for the popular audience, Sam Keen (1974) addressed the Apollonian and the Dionysian as the "rational" view and the "cosmic" view, respectively. He emphasized work as valued above play in the rational view, and the opposite value in the cosmic. In addition to this difference in content, work versus play, Keen suggested that in the rational view efficiency is sought, whereas in the cosmic view, it is ecstasy. The two world views can be summarized, as I understand Keen's position, as valuing efficient work (the rational or Apollonian view) or valuing ecstatic play (the cosmic or Dionysian view).

In his popular novel, *Zen and the Art of Motorcycle Maintenance,* Robert Pirsig (1974), too, addresses the Apollonian and Dionysian world views, naming them, respectively, "classical understanding" and "romantic understanding." His book is subtitled "an inquiry into values," and explores classical understanding and romantic understanding through what might well be seen as an allegory. The allegory involves riding and maintaining motorcycles on a long motorcycle journey. As he says, "Although motorcycle riding is romantic, motorcycle maintenance is purely classic" (Pirsig, 1974, p. 67). His exploration derives the following characterization of the classical understanding. Fundamentally, the world is seen as underlying form. From this, the mode of classical understanding proceeds in an orderly fashion using reason and laws or principles. Facts take priority over esthetic considerations, as thought takes priority over feelings in the pursuit of control.

Romantic understanding, for Pirsig, is derived from seeing the world in terms of immediate experience. Thus the mode of romantic understanding tends to be inspirational, imaginative, creative, and intuitive. Feelings and esthetic considerations are given priority over thoughts and facts in the pursuit of experience and intuitive understanding.

Of particular importance for the present essay is an insight offered by Pirsig concerning misunderstandings. He suggests that because persons tend to orient themselves through one of these two modes of understanding, classical *or* romantic, they will have difficulty understanding or appreciating those who orient through the other mode.

THE INSIGHT AND EXPRESSION POLARITY
IN PSYCHOTHERAPY

We see, then, that my opening quotes of Jack Nicholson and of William Blake reflect two different world views or value systems. Call them what you wish, keeping in mind that each pair of labels hints at a nuance of inflection: Apollonian-Dionysian, Logos-Eros, Rational-Cosmic, Classical-Romantic.

These two world views are manifest, as one might well expect, in the realm of psychotherapy. I suggest the terms "Insight" and "Expression" as the inflections in that realm. So, the Apollonian-Dionysian, Logos-Eros, Rational-Cosmic, Classical-Romantic world views and values are reflected in this microcosm as Insight-Expression psychotherapy views and values.

At this point, a side excursion is called for in the interest of clarifying the above idea of Insight-Expression in psychotherapy. In the 1960s, with a battle waging between behavior therapy and psychoanalysis, Perry London (1964) published a book which he titled *The Modes and Morals of Psychotherapy*. In this book, he distinguished two "modes," calling them "Insight Therapies" (meaning psychoanalysis, primarily) and "Action Therapies" (meaning behavior therapies). His thesis, as I understand him, was that Action Therapies are more appropriate for treating circumscribed symptoms and Insight Therapies are more appropriate for "expansion of consciousness." By way of implying the prescription of appropriate therapy to the problem–symptom or meaning of one's life–London appeared to have reached toward a truce between behavior therapy and psychoanalysis. He acknowledged the efficient control of symptoms such as phobias by means of behavior therapy. And, he acknowledged the legitimacy of exploring issues of meaning through psychoanalysis. He drew the distinction poignantly, and with poetic flair, when he queried rhetorically, "May not men leap from cliffs for other reasons than those for which dogs salivate to bells?" (London, 1964, p. 38).

Now, let us look at what London's writing suggests in light of the two world views. Action Therapies are designed for efficient control of symptoms, a goal-oriented task of mastery and molding, based on objective, unadorned technical application of underlying principles ("laws" of learning and conditioning). This is quite clearly a paragon of the Apollonian way.

But, what of Insight Therapies? London (p. 57) emphasized psychoanalysis as a way of raising consciousness. In psychoanalysis the emphasis is on *analyzing*. The taboo of "acting out" is based on the notion that if one acts on one's feelings, this interferes with analyzing their meaning. Not only does the acting out relieve one of the emotion, so it is no longer present for analysis, but psychic energy may be dissipated which could better have been used in the work of analysis. Thus, acting out can be a defense and a resistance. Psychoanalysis values insight, an intellectual task requiring reason. The traditional analyst was to be objective and apply precisely the psychoanalytic rules and techniques. Insight Therapies, as defined by London, are, I submit, more Apollonian than Dionysian. Perhaps not as extreme as Action Therapies, they are, nevertheless, basically an Apollonian approach. Analytic understanding of meaning is, indisputably, of the Logos. (Space does not permit me to garner here all of the evidence for my point. Keep in mind, I am referring to a classical psychoanalysis, not to some of the later developments which are under the rubric of "psychodynamic," or to some eclectic approaches which integrate psychodynamic theory or techniques with expressive therapies.)

Several years ago I was invited to be part of a "think-tank" for the National Institute of Mental Health. Our task was to derive guidelines for the funding of NIMH-sponsored research in the "experiential" psychotherapies. Perry London had been chosen to be the moderator. In the course of our discussions we struggled greatly with understanding each other and with agreeing on guidelines, or even agreeing on what experiential psychotherapy is. Looking back, I now see the difficulties as stemming largely from an Apollonian-Dionysian split. The good will, conscientiousness, and intellectual capability of all the participants was not adequate to overcome the difficulties completely. Most of the participants had, I see now, a strong Apollonian leaning, so to bring forth more Dionysian concerns tended to usher in confusion and frustration. And yet, the more Apollonian participants seemed fascinated with the Dionysian input. My impression is that Perry London, as well as the majority of the participants in the "think-tank," held an implicit Apollonian perspective, consistent with their expertise in Action or Insight Therapies.

Had Perry London been writing just a few years later, he perhaps would have included a third mode of therapy. To be complete, he would have to have included what are now identified as the Expressive Therapies. This mode includes Bioenergetics and other Neo-Reichian therapies (e.g., Core Energetics, Hakomi, Organismic Psychotherapy, Radix), Gestalt therapy, Pesso System Psychomotor therapy, Primal Scream therapy, and Psychodrama. Although some of these were being practiced at the time that London was writing, they really exploded onto the psychotherapy scene in the 1960s and 1970s. At the risk of oversimplification, I would characterize this mode as focusing on facilitating the person in therapy to open to creative and spontaneous expression of feelings.

To reiterate, then, my thesis is that the two competing world views are reflected in the realm of psychotherapy. Action Therapies (i.e., behavior therapies) are radically Apollonian. If we exclude them from our further discussion of *psycho*therapy, we can then see more clearly the dimension of Insight-Expression as the psychotherapy inflection of the Apollonian-Dionysian world views.

Let us now look more closely at the Insight mode of therapy as manifestation of the Apollonian world view. As I noted earlier, London emphasized,
using psychoanalysis as his major example, that Insight Therapies have as
their focus the raising of consciousness. (The meaning here is not in the sense
of "higher" consciousness as used in the context of transpersonal psychology, but rather in the sense of more thorough understanding.) As, too, I noted,
the focal activity of psychoanalysis is *analysis*. The purpose of psychoanalytic work is to analyze the life of the analysand, increasing understanding by
making functional connections between remembered childhood events and
feelings and current feelings, experiences and behaviors. With analysis
comes insight (Smith, 1999). Neurotic and characterological symptoms,
transference, dreams, and slips of the tongue all are part of the life of the
analysand and, as such, are grist for the analytic mill. "Thus, Freud wanted
analysands to *remember*, not escape from the unpleasantness of painful memories or the hard work of analysis by 'acting out' their issues" (Smith, 1999,
p. 75).

The Insight mode of therapy includes more than psychoanalysis. London
himself included Client-Centered therapy, making the claim that the distinction between interpretation (major tool of the analyst) and reflection (major
tool of the Client-Centered therapist) is more apparent than real. "The difference in usage is then a matter of exposing feelings in the proper context. The
Freudian requires more interpretive latitude in order to get them to appear in
the context of history, while the Rogerian can afford merely to reflect because
he will in any case interpret the exposed feeling with no reference to time"
(London, 1964, p. 50).

Elsewhere, I have suggested that Cognitive therapies also are of the Insight mode. "If taken in their broader meaning, and not restricted to their
technical psychoanalytic meaning, insight, interpretation, and analysis describe much of cognitive therapy as well as the myriad of psychodynamic
therapies. The essence is that the therapist is an external translator, tracing
things to their source and explaining to the person in therapy. Depending on
the proclivities of the therapist, the problems of living reported by the person
in therapy may be traced to [i.e., analyzed] childhood events or to irrational
beliefs and negative cognitive schemas . . . such analysis and explanation are
seen as *necessary* by psychodynamic and cognitive therapists alike" (Smith,
1999, p. 76).

So, the childhood event, the irrational belief, the negative cognitive sche-
ma, the unexposed feeling all constitute the "underlying form," the "unadorned fact," which is to be addressed "reasonably" ("objectively") and
"ordered" until "mastered." This is consonant with the Rational, the Classical, the Logos, the Apollonian.

In contrast, the Expressive mode of therapy honors the enactment of one's passion above the understanding of it. The various therapies which can be included under the Expressive rubric differ in the distance they place between the primary importance of expression and the secondary importance of understanding, but all look toward the ecstasy of passionate expression as their forte. They all value spontaneity in the surrender to feelings and immediate experience. All look to personal transformation, the metamorphosis for which Dionysus stands.

In the present writing I have referred to the Apollonian-Dionysian as a polarity or dimension. Horney (Shostrom, 1967), as noted earlier, saw them as two natural human tendencies, with no person being all one or all the other. So, too, it may be best to see Insight therapies and Expressive therapies as the poles of a continuum. Any given therapist may lean more one way or the other, as well, with the degree of leaning somewhat changeable. But for heuristic purposes it is easier, at times, to speak of the poles, not the continuum between. Thus, I identified the Insight mode of therapy as Apollonian and the Expressive mode as Dionysian. Additionally, at the extreme of the Apollonian pole is found the Action mode of therapy. At the extreme of the other pole, beyond the Dionysian lies the Bacchanalian. The Expressive mode, debased, is irresponsible and harmful, as some of us have witnessed, particularly in the excesses of the 1960s and 1970s. If the most extreme of the Expressive mode is Bacchanalian, with impulsive acting out and unbridled eros, what is the most extreme of the Action mode? It is dehumanization through the mechanical, dispassioned application of techniques. In the words of Paul Tillich (1962, p. 653), "A self which has become a matter of calculation and management has ceased to be a self. It has become a thing."

TOWARD A RESOLUTION OF THE POLARITY OF INSIGHT AND EXPRESSION

"Nothing too much." This was pithy advice of the Sages of Ancient Greece (Kopp, 1971). Applied to our topic, this could suggest not too much insight (meaning insight without expression), and not too much expression (meaning expression without insight). This sage advice is echoed in Aristotle's Doctrine of the Mean, popularly referred to as the "Golden Mean" (Popkin & Stroll, 1956). For Aristotle, this is the way to happiness, acting so as to steer a path between the two extremes. These ancient sources are a call to a resolution of polarities.

Both Insight Therapy and Expressive Therapy offer something of value, both have their forte, as we have already seen. But that valued emphasis, that strong point, may also be a limitation. Through the character of Harry Haller, known as the "Steppenwolf," Herman Hesse (1969, p. 55) demonstrates so clearly for us that ". . . every strength may become a weakness (and under some circumstances must). . . ." The poetic words of Jack Nicholson and of William Blake can now be read again, not just as messages of advocacy, but as messages of illumination. They elucidate "the weakness inherent in the strength" which Hesse addresses. We can paraphrase William Blake, making his point specific to psychotherapy: "Those who have Insight but do not give Expression to it, are creating deadness." For Jack Nicholson's words from *The Witches of Eastwick*, one might say: "Expression without benefit of Insight–the definition of 'impulsive' behavior–brings chaos to one's life."

We see, then, an emerging integration of Insight and Expression. Expression, the more liberal pole (that is, of Liber), animates and enlivens, celebrating aliveness. Insight, its guide, is the conservative pole, slowing the pace and lending security to each animated step. But, too much slowing of the pace may deaden, under the guise of security. "And you all know," Hecate (the lead witch in *Macbeth*) reminds us, "security is mortal's chiefest enemy" (Shakespeare, no year, p. 935).

If we turn, once again, to the mythopoetic, trusting in its metaphorical epistemology, we can be instructed in the relationship of Insight and Expression. The Norse god, Odin, appears in many hypostases including All-father, God of Poetry, God of the Dead, and God of Battle. As a shamanic figure, he was wont to shapeshift, taking on various forms in order to carry out his exploits. The many myths in which he has a part, often a leading role, show him to be passionate and active (Crossley-Holland, 1980).

We learn in the *Prose Edda* (Sturluson, 1954) that two ravens sit on the shoulders of Odin. He sends them out every day to fly over the whole world and return to him, bringing him news of all they see and hear. Their names are Hugin and Munin, meaning "Thought" and "Memory." Thus, we are told that Odin, active and passionate as he is, is informed by thought and memory. That is to say, Odin's Expression has benefit of Insight. Lee Hollander (1962, p. 57) in his translation of *The Poetic Edda*, speaks of Hugin and Munin as "'Thought' and 'Remembrance,' Othin's [sic] ravens which bring him intelligence."

At another level of interpretation, we can look to the birds themselves. They are ravens, seen in the Viking world as birds of the battle field. So, by virtue of the mental functions they stand for and the expressive activity they symbolize, they themselves are a metaphor for the bringing together of Insight and Expression.

Let us take the myth further. In *The Poetic Edda* (Hollander, 1962, p. 57) we find the following. "The whole earth over, every day, hover Hugin and Munin; I dread lest Hugin droop in his flight, yet I fear me still more for Munin." Is Odin telling us that he fears the loss of thought, but he fears the loss of memory more? It appears so. This would then suggest that the more conservative function (memory) is of the greater importance in the constitut-ing of guiding intelligence.

The Norse mythology, in summary, appears to offer us a clue to the reconciliation of the polarity of Insight and Expression. To wit, action is best guided when informed by thought *and* memory. Action/Expression, being liberal (i.e., of Liber) benefits from the conservative influence of thought and memory/Insight. Memory, being the more conservative, may be the more important component of Insight.

It was this Germanic/Norse mythology which served as cultural backdrop to the development of German philosophy. And, a case can be made that it was the nineteenth-century German philosophers, particularly Nietzsche, who provided the philosophical roots for the emerging psychologies of Freud, Jung, Adler, Rank, Reich, and in turn, Perls and Lowen. Of these luminaries, I believe it was Perls who best reflected the Odinic reconciliation of what in the psychotherapy context we call Insight and Expression. But, he did this in a manner which is decidedly Dionysian (Smith, 1991). Perhaps the Dionysian core of the Gestalt approach is best reflected by Arnold Beisser in his expression of the "paradoxical theory of change." Briefly stated, ". . . change occurs when one becomes what he is, not when he tries to become what he is not" (Beisser, 1970, p. 77). There it is, no mastery and control, but rather *the surrender to one's nature.*

Elsewhere, I have dealt in detail with Reich's system of therapy (Smith, 1985) and with Reich's influence on Perls in the development of Gestalt therapy (Smith, 1975, 1985). I will not take space to reiterate, except for specific points which are relevant in the remainder of the present essay.

My own approach to therapy is an integrative one, drawing heavily on the work of Reich and Perls, among others. I have described it in *The Body in Psychotherapy* (Smith, 1985) and in the book which Jeffrey Zeig and W. Michael Munion co-edited, *What Is Psychotherapy?* (Smith, 1990). My work is also presented in Richard Sharf's *Theories of Counseling and Psychothera-py* (1996, 2000).

In *The Body in Psychotherapy* (1985), I offer a model for the description and understanding of psychobiological existence based on need cycles, the cycles of contacting other people and other things in one's world for the satisfaction of needs and the withdrawal which follows. Calling this the Contact/Withdrawal Cycle, I explicate it in terms of natural and of pathologi-cal functioning. Space does not allow detail here. Put most briefly, the cycle consists of the arising of a Want, leading to organismic Arousal, which differentiates into Emotion, that calling for Action, which becomes an Inter-action with someone or something, which leads to Satisfaction of the Want. Following this Contact Episode comes Withdrawal until another Want be-comes figural, emerging from the background of potential Needs and Preferences. In the pathological form, there is self-interruption of the flow of the cycle through various pathological mechanisms serving to allow an avoidance of the next stage of the cycle.

Erring on the side of brevity, once more, I can summarize the "what," "why," and "how" of psychopathology as follows:

What is psychopathology? Any pattern of habitual self-interruption in the Contact/Withdrawal Cycle.

Why does one choose to self-interrupt? Self-interruptions are in response to a "toxic introject" (an introjected message which forbids full aliveness). The toxic introject consists of a content (what is specifically forbidden–the want, organismic Arousal or excitement, an Emotion, an Action, an Interaction, Satisfaction, Withdrawal, or some combination of these) and a "catastrophic expectation" (a threat that something catastrophic will happen if the voice of the toxic introject is disobeyed). So, the self-interruption is an avoidance of the next (forbidden) stage of the Contact/Withdrawal Cycle.

How can one self-interrupt? Self-interruptions are accomplished through a synergistic combination of four mechanisms: (1) Lowered Arousal through inadequate breathing; (2) Clouded Awareness through several means known in psychoanalysis as ego defense mechanisms; (3) Retroflected Action (action blocked or inhibited through "body armoring," i.e., chronic muscular tensions); (4) Retroflected Interaction (doing to oneself what one would like to do to the other or what one would like the other to do to one).

It is to the explication of the Contact/Withdrawal Cycle that much of *The Body in Psychotherapy* (Smith, 1985) is devoted. I leave it to the interested reader to consult this source if the details are desired. Hopefully, the overview just given will suffice for the purpose of the present essay.

My inspiration for the Contact/Withdrawal Cycle came primarily from the writings of Fritz Perls. From reading his books and articles, I became familiar with his idea that good contact requires both excitement and awareness. Consider this idea. Without excitement, or we could substitute "passion," contact with the environment will be weak and diminished. Good contact means satisfying contact, contact which satisfies some want. And, it implies action, but not just action per se, action which is interactive with someone or something. So, we have the notion of (passionate) action-interaction.

But the action-interaction sequence most often will miss the target, unless guided. The guide is "awareness." In the context of Gestalt therapy, "awareness" is preferred to the psychoanalytic term "insight." The former incorporates thought, memory, affect, and sensation, with particular emphasis on the senses. (Those of you who have traveled in Gestalt circles are familiar with the saying, "Lose your mind and come to your senses.") "Insight," in contrast, emphasizes thought and memory, with particular emphasis on memory.

Awareness is the guide–awareness of one's Want (both need and preference, given options for meeting that need), awareness of Arousal (excitement), awareness of Emotion (passion), awareness of Satisfaction. What is guided is Action-Interaction, the Expressive portion of the Contact Episode. So, we see an intimate link of interdependence between Awareness and Expression.

Erving Polster (1970, p. 70) in his typically thoughtful and clear manner wrote, ". . . knowing the difference between being hungry, angry, or sexually aroused surely is a lengthy step toward knowing what to do. In this interplay between feeling and doing lies the crux of our search for good living." Using the metaphor of the synaptic arc which facilitates union between sensory and motor neurons, he introduced the concept of the "synaptic experience." By this he meant the experience of union between awareness and expression. Furthermore, Polster suggested that some people are more "awareness oriented," some more "action oriented."

I see the "synaptic experience" as a core value in the Gestalt approach, as well as a core concept. In the inimitable style of Zen, with its paradox of simplicity and profundity, a story is told. When a jealous competitor challenged a Priest named Bankei, trying to show that he had no miraculous powers, and holding up yet another priest as greater, Bankei replied, "Perhaps your fox can perform that trick, but that is not the manner of Zen. My miracle is that when I feel hungry I eat and when I feel thirsty I drink" (Reps, no date, p. 68). The real miracle–"consciousness in action" (p. 175).

If we look at Apollo and Bacchus as representing the extremes of the poles, then Dionysus represents a moderated position (relative to Bacchus). As a therapy which follows the Dionysian path (Smith, 1991), Gestalt therapy is, then, not extreme. It is, however, decidedly Dionysian in its emphasis on Expression as pre-eminent.

One of the ways in which Expression is ascendent in the Gestalt approach is illustrated in the Contact/Withdrawal Cycle. There are feedback loops in the cycle such that later steps clarify and enhance earlier steps. "For example, taking action may enhance the felt emotion, or if the action is not appropriate to the emotion, the action may reveal to the person what the actual emotion would be if it were allowed into awareness. It is as if there were a reverberating wave which further enhances previous steps as each new step is taken" (Smith, 1985, p. 31). In practice, this means that often the person in therapy is encouraged to express (Action-Interaction) in a psychodramatic way in the therapy session as a means of discovering or clarifying an underlying Emotion, Arousal, or Want. In other words, Awareness may emerge from Expression. As Hugh Prather wrote (1970, no page number), "Sometimes the only way for me to find out what it is I want to do is to go ahead and do something. Then the moment I start to act, my feelings become clear."

Insight therapies, especially more psychoanalytic ones, tend to take the path of: talking → memories (thinking) → feelings. In contrast, an Expressive therapy, such as my body-oriented Gestalt approach, offers the alternative path of: body work → feelings → memories. The body work may consist of a variety of techniques, as discussed in *The Body in Psychotherapy* (Smith, 1985), in addition to psychodramatic expressive work. These techniques include selected body postures, gentle touching, "catalytic touch" (Brown, 1990), directed breathing, Bioenergetic "stress postures" (Lowen & Lowen, 1977), "orgonomic massage" (Reich, 1949), and so forth. The key, here, is that feelings are directly accessed through body experience and expression.

The idea in the Gestalt approach is that Awareness and Expression are themselves two parts of a Gestalt. As parts of a Gestalt, they cannot be fully understood in isolation, but only in their relationship. Speaking wistfully, Barry Stevens (1984, p. 4) asks, "What is it but awareness and acting in accord with circumstances?" Yes, awareness *and* acting, Awareness and Expression. She wrote further, emphasizing the integrity of this Gestalt, "Observation/understanding/action without an intervening period of thought" (Stevens, 1984, p. 85). This same integrity is reflected in Gestalt praxis when Fritz Perls (1998, p. 72) instructs us that "The reintegration of the dissociated parts of the personality is best undertaken by resensitizing and remobilizing the symptoms of orientation and manipulation." He is calling attention to both resensitizing desensitized orientation functions, that is, Awareness, *and* remobilizing frozen Expression. Borrowing from Everett Shostrom (1967), I have suggested to therapists in training with me a simple guide for working with persons in therapy. It can be used as a reminder to facilitate the process of the person in therapy. "*Identify* feeling, *experience* the feeling, *express* the feeling." Again, the Gestalt of Awareness *and* Expression.

In the Gestalt approach, then, we find the resolution of the polarity of Insight and Expression. We need only to translate the more historically bound concept of insight into the more here-and-now focused concept of lived (experienced) Awareness. Awareness and Expression, then, represent two parts of a whole, two parts of a Gestalt. (In the Contact/Withdrawal Cycle, they are further differentiated into smaller constituent parts Want, Arousal, Emotion, Satisfaction and Action, Interaction, respectively.) In spontaneous living, Awareness flows into Expression. They are wed as one.

AWE AND TERROR IN THE EXPERIENCE OF THE GESTALT OF AWARENESS AND EXPRESSION

My introduction to body work was at a Summer Workshop of the American Academy of Psychotherapists. Vivian Guze, who had trained with both Fritz Perls and Alexander Lowen, was offering a workshop on Bioenergetics.

When she asked for a demonstration volunteer, preferably one who was not experienced with Bioenergetics, I came forward. I was both curious and naive. Vivian asked me to bend backwards over a "breathing stool," a backless bar stool with a rolled-up blanket on it, with the center of my back on the mid-point of the stool. Following the instructions of her soft voice, I placed my arms back over my head, letting them dangle, dropped my chin, and made an a-a-a-h-h sound with each exhalation. From time to time, she placed her hand along my sternum and made a firm vibratory motion directed downward into my chest as I exhaled. What I experienced was awesome. I felt a rush of aliveness throughout my body, or more accurately, throughout my whole being. The level of energy which I felt was intense, almost more than I thought I could handle. Vivian's confident and calm voice helped me not to panic, although I had moments of fear as the feeling of energy pulsed in me. My sounds grew louder, perhaps they were screams. Then, Vivian invited me to stand up slowly, and then, once I had my feet solidly under me, once I was well "grounded," to bend forward with knees slightly bent, allowing my arms and head to hang. This position balanced the previous position of a back bend over the stool. What I noticed when I stood up, finally, was that my vision was unusually clear, colors were very vivid, and my voice, when I spoke, sounded deeper and more resonant than how I remembered it. I felt warm and very good, a rather paradoxical excited calmness. This transformation, occurring in just a few minutes, I later estimated, was dramatic. I was so awed by my experience that I knew I wanted to learn body-oriented psychotherapy. I also knew that I was not ready to pursue this powerful level of work yet. It was fully a year before I began my training in Bioenergetics. During that year I read about the approach and continued in my personal therapy which was Insight oriented.

What is so awesome, so terrifying about waking up, coming alive? In describing my integrative approach, I wrote, "It is the exquisite focus on organism-in-environment *process* which appeals most to me about the Gestalt approach. To this I add the awesome power of the Reichian and neo-Reichian procedures for assessing and facilitating that process" (Smith, 1985, p. ix). Gestalt may be characterized as a therapy which focuses on personal process as that unfolds moment by moment in the here-and-now of the therapy session. In the unfolding of personal process, as reflected in the tracking of the Contact/Withdrawal Cycle, the self-interruption becomes apparent. As the person in therapy flows through a cycle, the usually abrupt self-interruption bespeaks an avoidance. The avoidance is of the next step, the step in the unfolding process which is forbidden by the toxic introject. By bumping into the toxic introject, specifically with confronting the catastrophic expectation, anxiety is aroused. As Perls (1998, p. 90) said in an early session, only more recently published as a paper, "Any emotion that is not developed as emotion will appear as anxiety. It's the blocking of the natural flow of vitality." And, of course, by "not developed" he meant the avoidance of the expression of that emotion. So, moving ahead with natural process, in spite of a catastrophic expectation, can be terrifying. In this context, Erving and Miriam Polster (1973, p. 119) have written that ". . . change itself calls forth terror. . . ." When one has done so and discovered the catastrophe did not ensue, the experience can be awesome.

In the growth toward natural, spontaneous expression there is a particularly troublesome stage which is frequently encountered. In introducing this, the Polsters wrote of four levels of expression: blocked, inhibited, exhibitionistic, and spontaneous. The blocked and inhibited stages are both non-expressive. In the case of the former, the person does not know what he or she wants to express and in the latter, the person knows, but expresses not. The third stage, the exhibitionistic, is reached when the person does express what he or she wants, but the expression is new. Not yet fully integrated or assimilated into the personality, expression at the exhibitionistic stage may be awkward. But, as the Polsters (1973, p. 126) pointed out, ". . . one does not simply and uniformly move into grace from a blocked or inhibited position. . . . Some willingness to accept the . . . awkward moments is indispensable to growth." I would add that with the awkwardness of the exhibitionistic stage may also come terror.

In words and description more in keeping with the awe and terror of which we are speaking, Wilhelm Reich (1949) posited what he called a "phase of the breakdown of secondary narcissism." Reich suggested that the continuing frustration of natural needs leads to contraction of the body armor (chronic muscular tensions). It is this conflict between inhibited impulses and the inhibiting armor that leads to a secondary narcissism (as contrasted with the primary narcissism which results when the infant cathects her or his own body parts as part-objects of love). In other words, as investment of libido in the outside world is made more difficult or is withdrawn, the energy builds up within, intensifying a secondary narcissism. When the armor, which is the characterological protective mechanism, is loosened or dissolved, there is a temporary condition of helplessness. This is the phase of the breakdown of secondary narcissism. During this phase, the person has strong, freed energy, but with a concomitant lack of "safe" neurotic controls. This phase of therapy is often stormy, with the person feeling terror.

Perls probably borrowed from Reich's phase of the breakdown of secondary narcissism, including the essence of it in his five layer model of neurosis (Smith, 1975a). Although consistent in his conceptual presentation of the layers of neurosis, he was not always consistent in his numbering of them. Disregarding the numbering, then, the layers emerge as follows (Smith, 1985): Neurosis is characterized by a *cliche layer*, a layer of tokens of meaning. Beneath that is a layer of playing roles, playing "games," a *phony layer.* Next is the *impasse layer,* characterized by the "phobic attitude." At this phobic layer the phobic attitude results in avoidance of contact, and in turn, the feeling of being lost, empty, stuck, and confused. Beneath this is the death layer or *implosive layer* where the person is paralyzed by opposing forces, trying to pull in and hold herself or himself together. If successfully worked through, this implosive layer will unfold into the final layer, the *explosive layer.*

The explosive layer is characterized by authentic experiencing and expression of emotion. The explosion may be into grief, if a loss had not been assimilated, or joy, or anger, or sexual feelings. There is a clear parallel, here, between Reich's phase of the breakdown of secondary narcissism and Perls' progression through the impasse, to implosion, and to explosion. The essence in both cases is the dissolution of organismic core defenses in order to emerge, after the "walk through hell," with an authentic expression. The impasse, for Perls (1969), is the position where environmental support or obsolete inner support is no longer adequate and authentic self-support has not yet been achieved. Staying with the experience of the impasse, enduring the hell of confusion and helplessness, leads to growth. If one will but stay with her or his techniques of self-interruption (avoidance), experiencing the attendant confusion to the utmost, she or he may experience something like a hypnogogic hallucination, a blinding flash of insight. I am reminded, here, of a quote from Proust, "To heal a suffering one must experience it to the full" (Beisser, 1970, p. 78). And so the surrender, and so the terror. And, so the awe!

I want to add a brief discussion of methodology. Gestalt methods or techniques may be understood by viewing them as involving either *concentration* or *presentification,* both of which are in the service of creating the *here-and-now experience* (Smith, 1975b, 1978). Presentification, a term suggested by Claudio Naranjo (1970), refers to enactment in the present, the bringing of unfinished business from the past or fantasies of the future into this moment for psychodramatic expression. By so doing, a psychologically real event is created and experienced, as opposed to a "distantiated" (kept at a distance) event talked about in the "there-and-then."

The vividness of the here-and-now experience may be increased by the several techniques of concentration. "Con-centra-tion," being with the center of the experience, involves making the perceptual figure more prominent, and the perceptual ground or background less prominent. The psychodrama may be vivified by means of slowing down. Awareness takes time to develop, and so may be increased when the pace is slowed. Just as slowing down increases the time spent in the experience, repeating allows multiple exposures as another way of increasing that time. Sometimes, particularly if the meaning of an experience is not clear, exaggeration of the expression will make the meaning obvious. Contrasting an expression with its opposite may also clarify its meaning, so shuttling between the two may be useful. These several Gestalt techniques–slowing down, repeating a behavior, exaggerating a behavior, and shuttling between the behavior and its opposite–all are ways of creating greater vividness of experience, and are often used in the psycho-drama of presentification.

Making the background less vivid serves to make it less distracting, taking less away from the vividness of the focal experience in the psychodrama. This is done by minimizing environmental distractions or "noise" from the therapy setting. It also involves facilitating the person in therapy to identify and not do those things which he or she may be doing to distract himself or herself (e.g., thinking about something irrelevant in order to avoid a feeling).

Through skillful and artistic use of the techniques of presentification and concentration, the therapist facilitates the creation of a vivid here-and-now experience, a taste of full presence. As personal process unfolds moment by moment, a psychodrama is created, and more or less elaborated, constituting a psychologically real experience. By honoring the flow of fully embodied Awareness into fully embodied Expression, full, natural aliveness may be born. The limited aliveness of the past may be reframed. Analogous to "cog-nitive reframing," this is a "conative reframing" (reframing in action), in-volving not the limited Insight of the former, but a Gestalt of Awareness and Insight.

As we have seen, Reich and Perls in similar terms have warned of the storm, the walk through hell. Awesome in its power for awakening to alive-ness, yet terrifying in the departure from the safety of Apollonian mastery and control, the embodied Gestalt approach honors the Dionysian. And still, in its surrender to the inspiration and ecstasy of immediate experience, there lurks the danger of drift into Bacchanalian excess. But, as a more recent Greek by the name of Zorba said (through the mouth of Anthony Quinn),

A man needs a little madness,
or else . . . he never dares
cut the rope and be free.

REFERENCES

Beisser, A. (1970). The paradoxical theory of change. In J. Fagan & I. Shepherd (Eds.), *Gestalt therapy now* (pp. 77-80). Palo Alto, CA: Science and Behavior Books.

Brown, M. (1990). *The healing touch: An introduction to Organismic Psychotherapy.* Mendocino, CA: Life Rhythm.

Campbell, J. (1990). *Transformations of myth through time.* New York: Harper & Row.

Crossley-Holland, K. (1980). *The Norse myths.* New York: Pantheon.

Funk & Wagnalls standard dictionary of folklore, mythology, and legend. (1984). New York: Harper & Row.

Hamilton, E. (1942). *Mythology.* New York: Mentor.

Hesse, H. (1969). *Steppenwolf.* New York: Bantam.

Hollander, L. (Translator). (1962). *The Poetic Edda.* Austin, TX: University of Texas Press.

Jung, C. (1970). *Civilization in transition.* Princeton, NJ: Princeton University Press.

Kaufmann, W. (Ed.). (1982). *The portable Nietzsche.* New York: Viking Penguin.

Keen, S. (1974). The cosmic versus the rational. *Psychology Today, 8* (2), 56-59.

Kierkegaard, S. (1993). *The diary of Soren Kierkegaard.* (Edited by Peter Rohde). Secaucus, NJ: Carol.

Kopp, S. (1971). *Guru.* Palo Alto, CA: Science and Behavior Books.

Lewis, C. S. (1996). *The Screwtape letters.* New York: Touchstone.

London, P. (1964). *The modes and morals of psychotherapy.* New York: Holt, Rinehart, and Winston.

Lowen, A. & Lowen, L. (1977). *The way to vibrant health.* New York: Harper & Row.

Naranjo, C. (1970). Present-centeredness: Technique, prescription, and ideal. In J. Fagan & I. Shepherd (Eds.), *Gestalt therapy now* (pp. 47-69). Palo Alto, CA: Science and Behavior Books.

Partridge, B. (1960). *A history of orgies.* New York: Bonanza.

Perls, F. (1969). *Gestalt therapy verbatim.* Moab, UT: Real People Press.

Perls, F. (1998). The manipulator: A session of Gestalt therapy with Dr. Frederick Perls and group. *The Gestalt Journal, 21* (2), 75-90.

Pirsig, R. (1974). *Zen and the art of motorcycle maintenance.* New York: William Morrow.

Polster, E. (1970). Sensory functioning in psychotherapy. In J. Fagan & I. Shepherd (Eds.), *Gestalt therapy now* (pp. 70-76). Palo Alto, CA: Science and Behavior Books.

Polster, E. & Polster, M. (1973). *Gestalt therapy integrated.* New York: Brunner Mazel.

Popkin, R. & Stroll, A. (1956). *Philosophy made simple.* Garden City, NY: Doubleday.

Prather, H. (1970). *Notes to myself.* New York: Bantam.

Prather, H. (1972). *I touch the earth, the earth touches me.* Garden City, NY: Doubleday.

Reich, W. (1949). *Character analysis.* New York: Noonday Press.

Reps, p. (Compiler). (no date). *Zen flesh, Zen bones.* Garden City, NY: Anchor.

Sabin, F. (1940). *Classical myths that live today.* New York: Silver Burdett.

Shakespeare, W. (no year). Macbeth. In *The complete works of William Shakespeare* (pp. 922-944). Cleveland, OH: World Syndicate.

Sharf, R. (1996, 2000). *Theories of psychotherapy and counseling.* Belmont, CA: Brooks/Cole.

Shostrom, E. (1967). *Man, the manipulator.* Nashville, TN: Abingdon.

Smith, E. (1975a). The role of early Reichian theory in the development of Gestalt therapy. *Psychotherapy: Theory, Research and Practice, 12* (3), 268-272.

Smith, E. (1975b). Altered states of consciousness in Gestalt therapy. *Journal of Contemporary Psychotherapy, 7* (1), 35-40.

Smith, E. (1978). The impasse phenomenon: A Gestalt therapy experience involving an altered state of consciousness. *The Gestalt Journal, 1* (1), 88-93.

Smith, E. (1985). *The body in psychotherapy.* Jefferson, NC: McFarland.

Smith, E. (1990). Embodied Gestalt psychotherapy. In J. Zeig & W. Munion (Eds.), *What is psychotherapy?* (pp. 107-111). San Francisco: Jossey-Bass.

Smith, E. (1991). Gestalt, a Dionysian path. *Voices, 14* (2), 61-69.

Smith, E. (1999). Enactment and awareness in the Gestalt approach. *Voices, 35* (4), 74-77.

Stevens, B. (1984). *Burst out laughing.* Berkeley, CA: Celestial Arts.

Sturluson, S. (1954). *Prose Edda.* (Translated by Jean Young). Berkeley, CA: University of California Press.

Tillich, p. (1962). The courage to be. In W. Barrett & H. Aiken (Eds.), *Philosophy in the twentieth century* (pp. 652-687). New York: Random House.

Standing in Awe:
The Cosmic Dimensions
of Effective Psychotherapy

Kirk J. Schneider

SUMMARY. This article presents a personal reflection on therapeutic awe. Formally, I define awe as the co-mingling of humility, reverence, and wonder before creation; informally, I understand it as the thrill and anxiety of living. Awe is not spotlighted very often as a therapeutic "condition," but in my work and that of many of my colleagues it is the sine qua non of healing. In this article, I examine the nature, role, and salutary implications of therapeutic awe. Two brief cases are provided to illustrate. *[Article copies available for a fee from The Haworth Document Delivery Service: 1-800-342-9678. E-mail address: <getinfo@haworthpressinc. com> Website: <http://www.HaworthPress.com> © 2001 by The Haworth Press, Inc. All rights reserved.]*

KEYWORDS. Mystery, avoidance, systems, drugs, multiplicity, wisdom, elasticity, healing, suffering, wonder

---

Kirk J. Schneider is a psychologist in private practice in San Francisco, CA, where he is a co-founder and current president of the Existential-Humanistic Institute. He serves on the editorial boards of *The Psychotherapy Patient*, the *Journal of Humanistic Psychology*, and the *Review of Existential Psychology and Psychiatry*. He is an adjunct faculty member at Saybrook Graduate School and the Calif. Institute for Integral Studies. His books include *The Paradoxical Self* (1990), *Horror and the Holy* (1993), and, co-authored with Rollo May, *The Psychology of Existence: An Integrative, Clinical Perspective* (1995). His current project is *The Handbook of Humanistic Psychology* (in press), of which he is senior editor.

Address correspondence to: Kirk J. Schneider, PhD, 1738 Union Street, San Francisco, CA 94123 (E-mail: kschneider@california.com).

[Haworth co-indexing entry note]: "Standing in Awe: The Cosmic Dimensions of Effective Psychotherapy." Schneider, Kirk J. Co-published simultaneously in *The Psychotherapy Patient* (The Haworth Press, Inc.) Vol. 11, No. 3/4, 2001, pp. 123-127; and: *Frightful Stages: From the Primitive to the Therapeutic* (ed: Robert B. Marchesani, and E. Mark Stern) The Haworth Press, Inc., 2001, pp. 123-127. Single or multiple copies of this article are available for a fee from The Haworth Document Delivery Service [1-800-342-9678, 9:00 a.m. - 5:00 p.m. (EST). E-mail address: getinfo@haworthpressinc.com].

123

No one who has not experienced how insubstantial the pageant of external reality can be, how it may fade, can fully realize the sublime and grotesque presences that can replace it, or that can exist along side it.

-R.D. Laing (1967, p. 133)

INTRODUCTION

The awesomeness of life is the starting point for psychology. Any psychology worth its name must begin with this premise.

By awesomeness, I mean first of all mystery–incomprehensibility, unmanageability; and second of all, fascination, bedazzlement. I am not simply speaking here of the sentiment we experience when we gaze at stars; I am speaking of the brute awareness that we exist at all.

Awe is not a very comfortable standpoint for many people. (It certainly was not for the biblical Job!) Hence, all about us today, we see avoidance of awe–by burying ourselves in materialist science, for example, or in absolutist religious positions; or by locking ourselves into systems, whether corporate, familial, or consumerist; or by stupefying ourselves with drugs. We also, ironically, see the avoidance of awe in positions that profess to embrace life's multiplicity. Some postmodernists, for example, imply that awe is a historical or cultural artifact, as profound or significant as any other historical or cultural perspective.

More than ever before, it seems to me, we are in need of the wisdom that awe inspires. We are in need of paradoxical wisdom. We need to see the complexity of things, the wholeness of things, which means the incompleteness and simplicity of things at the same time. We need to see that as soon as we polarize, we partialize our understanding. As soon as we fixate, even if we fixate on what appears to be open and multiple, we lose the vitality of our being, the elasticity of our being, and the poignant predicament of our being.

This article explores the role and implications of an "awe-based" psychotherapy. My main thesis is that an awe-inspired attitude derives from deep and foundation-shaking experiences in life and is a prerequisite to optimal existential therapy. Further, awe opens the therapist's understanding of both the client's struggle as well as potential for healing into the context of the self-cosmic relation. The relation to the cosmic or being is a specter, as I view it, that haunts virtually the entire spectrum of so-called psychopathologies. For example, for many, the experience of depression is not just an experience of smallness and insignificance before the local context of family or vocation, but a sense of smallness and insignificance before being itself (the mysterium tremendum). The fundamental experience of healing, on the other hand, also greatly exceeds the circumscribed world of symptoms, family, or vocation, but relates to one's entire engagement with life. In the final part of my paper, I will provide two brief cases to illustrate the foregoing.

FROM NORMALITY TO AWE

Suffering is not an issue of dysregulation. Health is not a matter of self-regulation. Dysregulation and regulation equal the medicalization of experience. The medicalization of experience implies a standard of "normal" vs. "abnormal" brain functioning. Did the Nazi functionaries at the Nuremberg War Crime Trials have "normal" brains? Did the "intelligensia" who complied with Aryan propaganda or the Witch Trials in Salem or the Inquisition in Spain, have "normal" brains? What about John Q. Public who engages in the same dull jobs and relationships, over and over again–how "normal" is his brain? And what of the pill-popping day trader, the beer-guzzling sports fanatic, or the steel-jawed executive officer–are they the "norms" that are so coveted today?

As psychotherapists, we are all social advocacy agents. The question is what form of society do we advocate? Do we advocate social adjustment, reflexive accommodation? Or do we advocate liberation, the demystification of "normalcy," awe? Personally, I've had enough of the normalization program; from here on I'm an "awe-advocacy agent."

The problem with our competency-based therapy is our competency-based culture. So much is geared to the aggregate, the programmable, the saleable. The conventional message is: Engage in therapy, not to open up, not to discover, not to find a passion in life, but to stay out of trouble, to fit in, to conform to the needs of the mass-market. The "revolving door" of psychotherapy is rampant today. Why? Because conventional therapy fails to cultivate trust; it fails to encourage self-reflection; and it fails to provide time. The net result of these failures is that inner struggle, the seed of substantive healing for many people, is almost completely overlooked. That which is conventionally attended to, on the other hand, is a drug or program that thoroughly bypasses the life affirming/negating battles out of which profound illumination can occur. And while a person may be changed by such a regimen, he will not likely experience himself as the core or agent of that change. As a result, he will wither.

There is a great need in our world to move from normalizing and fitting in to opening up and finding out, from "competency" based education to awe-based education, and from social advocacy to awe advocacy. In the balance of this article, I will ponder my experience as an awe advocacy agent. First I will define awe, then I will trace its implications for suffering and healing.

AWE: A DEFINITION

Awe is awesome, it is awful. The stakes in awe are cosmic. When one is awed, the localized is dashed; fear becomes anxiety, trauma terror, and healing holiness. Formally, I define awe as humility, reverence, and wonder before creation; informally, I view it as the thrill and anxiety of living. Awe is humbling because it is a realization of the mysterium tremendum (Otto, 1923)–or inscrutable mystery–of every moment. Awe is reverential because in addition to inspiring humility and dread, it also sparks adoration, admiration, and appreciation. Finally, awe inspires wonder–a sense of both amazement and curiosity.

SUFFERING AND AWE

The stakes in suffering are cosmic. Consider the process of breakdown. In a breakdown or crisis, there is a crack in the protective shell of consciousness, a rent in the fabric of identity. The shock of radical change opens one to both the terror and beauty of creation; the inertia of sameness, on the other hand, dulls one from such a sensibility. It is a curious irony of life that whatever traumatizes also potentially liberates, and whatever consoles also potentially deadens. "Where danger is," wrote Holderlin in Patmos, "the delivering power also grows."

The cracking of the cosmic egg leads to awesome new sensations, feelings, and thoughts. That which we formerly took for granted, a loved one, our health, a quiescent mind, shatters; that which emerges stuns. Suffering opens us to the primal forces, emotions, blood, upheaval. Where safety once permeated, now we must fend for ourselves; where a smile once warmed us, now there is a cold abyss. Or, as so many clients convey, "the bottom has dropped out" and "the world has collapsed." Yet the climb back up or the re-collecting of pieces is not without reward. It is here that we arrive at the multidimensionality of suffering–the depths and the heights of aliveness–that no "average" consciousness can match. If we can but stay present to it, the process of suffering informs us, not just of our passing and "microbial" nature, but of a nature yet to be discovered.

AWE IN PSYCHOTHERAPY

As a therapist, I often have the sense of being on an enormous collaborative journey with my clients. Indeed, to one of my clients, I am "Captain Kirk." While many therapists are struck by their clients' words, it is my clients' eyes, mouths, and bodies that strike me. It is their movement, their positioning, and their manner that captivate me, not so much the individual things they say. While the individual things that clients say are indeed important–and sometimes must be focused upon–rarely are they as urgent, compelling, or essential as the process or presence by which those statements are made. And it is precisely here that awe is necessitated. It is precisely in the space of awe that the cosmic proportion of clients' battles is illuminated–the abject terror and the tenacious rage; the torrential grief and the persistent hope; all else is sacrilege.

Without awe, my clients cannot substantively experience themselves. Without experiencing themselves, my clients languish.

Severely abused as a child and young wife, M was always informing me of the latest horror classic at the local theater. She sent me "Godzilla" stamps on her letters, and showed me books about death.

M was intimate with shadows. Her whole life had been sorrowful. But through it all were the seeds of awe. As abominable as her suffering had been, as extreme as her torment, there were also glimpses of the marvelous–ghosts, archetypes, raptures–in her ordeals. These were glimpses not afforded those of "normal" lineage. With awe as a guiding medium, I invited M to grapple with these wildly oscillating rifts within herself and eventually (through massive toil), to bridge and transform them.

Karen too was a sufferer. Her torment was overeating. "I went from an angry mother to an angry God to being angry at myself," declared Karen (Roth, 1991, p. 181). After three-and-a-half years of sustained therapy, however, Karen echoed M: "Now I am living. . . . Last week at work, I saw some bare oak trees covered with raindrops. I knew they were just raindrops on a naked tree, but to me they were diamonds" (pp. 180, 183).

She concluded:

> I wish I could tell you that being a size twelve is all wonderful but I'm finding out that being awake and alive is a package deal. I don't get to go through the line and pick only goodies. On one side is wonder, awe, excitement and laughter–and on the other side is tears, disappointment, aching sadness. Wholeness is coming to me by being willing to explore ALL the feelings. (p. 183-184)

A more compelling case for therapeutic awe could hardly be formulated.

REFERENCES

Laing, R.D. (1967). *Politics of experience.* New York: Ballantine.
Otto, R. (1923). *The idea of the holy.* New York: Oxford University Press.
Roth, G. (1991). *When food is love.* New York: Plume.

You Will Have These Awe-Full Moments When You Have Your Own Experiential Session

Alvin R. Mahrer

SUMMARY. There are three moments of awe that seem to occur in each experiential session. Although these sessions can occur with an experiential teacher-therapist, the emphasis is on having one's own experiential session. Each experiential session is designed to go through a prescribed series of steps. When the steps are followed carefully, a generally regular consequence is the occurrence of the three moments of awe. Each of these three awe-full moments is described in some detail. *[Article copies available for a fee from The Haworth Document Delivery Service: 1-800-342-9678. E-mail address: <getinfo@haworthpressinc.com> Website: <http://www.HaworthPress.com> © 2001 by The Haworth Press, Inc. All rights reserved.]*

KEYWORDS. Transformation, change, experiencing, life scenes, silliness, zaniness, exhilaration, conversion, fascination, anguish, terror

The purpose of this article is to describe experiential sessions that almost everyone can carry out by themselves, and the awe-full moments that usually occur in these experiential sessions. The purpose of the article following this one is to illustrate what it was like for one person to go through the awe-full moments in one of his own experiential sessions. The purpose of this and the

Alvin R. Mahrer, PhD, is affiliated with the School of Psychology, University of Ottawa, Ottawa, Ontario, Canada K1N 6N5 (E-mail: amahrer@uottawa.ca).

[Haworth co-indexing entry note]: "You Will Have These Awe-Full Moments When You Have Your Own Experiential Session." Mahrer, Alvin R. Co-published simultaneously in *The Psychotherapy Patient* (The Haworth Press, Inc.) Vol. 11, No. 3/4, 2001, pp. 129-140; and: *Frightful Stages: From the Primitive to the Therapeutic* (ed: Robert B. Marchesani, and E. Mark Stern) The Haworth Press, Inc., 2001, pp. 129-140. Single or multiple copies of this article are available for a fee from The Haworth Document Delivery Service [1-800-342-9678, 9:00 a.m. - 5:00 p.m. (EST). E-mail address: getinfo@haworthpressinc.com].

following article is to invite you to take a step toward having your own experiential session and going through these awe-full moments.

EXPERIENTIAL SESSIONS CAN OCCUR BY ONESELF OR WITH AN EXPERIENTIAL TEACHER-THERAPIST

Consider two different pictures of what is meant by experiential sessions. In one picture, you are alone in a room. You have the skills to go through an experiential session by yourself. You know what to do and how to do it. You are the "practitioner." Throughout the session, you are in a large comfortable chair with your feet on a comfortable footrest, or perhaps you are lying on a bed. Your eyes are closed throughout the entire session, which usually lasts for an hour and a half or so, sometimes an hour, sometimes two hours. No one is around to disturb you or even to hear you going through the whole session by yourself. This is one picture of an experiential session.

In a different picture, you are in the office of an experiential teacher-therapist. The office is likely sound-proof. A large part of the teacher's job is to show you how to be able to have a session by yourself, and to do this by going through the steps of the session along with you. Accordingly, to do this, and especially for the teacher to be able to attend to what you attend to, the two chairs are close alongside each other, both facing in the same direction. Both of you have your eyes closed throughout the entire session which also lasts for about one to two hours, ending when the work is done or when both of you agree that the session is over.

The experiential teacher-therapist guides you through the session, showing you what to do next and how to do it, depending on your proficiency, and also joins right with you in undergoing what you are undergoing as you proceed through the session. The session moves along at your own personal pace, honoring your own readiness and willingness to go through each step, however small. This is the second picture of what is meant by an experiential session.

Whether the experiential sessions are with yourself or with an experiential teacher-therapist, you can have experiential sessions throughout your life. Picture your having sessions throughout your whole life. If the sessions are by yourself, you probably have sessions on a rather regular basis, for example, every week or two, or whenever you want to have a session. If the session is with an experiential teacher-therapist, you can have sessions whenever you wish, successively or spread out, with varying periods in between sessions. You may start having sessions whenever you wish, as young or as old as you are. I seem to have experiential sessions every few weeks or less.

You probably do not need any special qualities to be able to have your own experiential sessions. There seem to be no special talents or expertise or qualities you need to have your own experiential sessions. You do not have to be a loner, a do-it-yourselfer, psychologically sophisticated, someone who has been in psychotherapy, someone with knowledge about the psyche or inner world. You can be young or old, a tower of strength or rusted out hulk, someone who has rarely tried to probe inside or someone whose life was spent digging inside your own thoughts and feelings. Just about everyone can have his or her own experiential sessions.

You probably do not need any special qualities to be able to have the awe-full moments. The awe-full moments come with the sessions. In other words, as you follow the steps and the methods of going through an experiential session, you will be brought face-to-face with some awe-full moments. These awe-full moments will tend to occur because you are doing a good job of going through the session, not because of any special qualities you may have.

These particular awe-full moments will tend to happen whether you have had lots of experiences of awe or practically none at all, whether there is something a little dreamy about you or you are more of a hard-reality sort of person, whether you are artistic or not especially, whether you are religious and spiritual or not much at all.

WHEN YOU HAVE YOUR OWN EXPERIENTIAL SESSION, THE GOAL IS TO BECOME THE PERSON YOU ARE CAPABLE OF BECOMING, AND TO BE FREE OF THE PAINFUL SCENE-SITUATION

Each experiential session offers the person opportunity after opportunity to go beyond the point of no return in hurling oneself into the awe-full final leap. Each experiential session has a series of invitations to a series of final leaps. The goals of each experiential session invite the person to take these momentous final leaps.

The goals and the in-session steps are not aimed at putting the person in some sort of state of awe, or at putting the person through moments of awe. However, if the person has an eye on the goals, and if the person actually walks through the steps, one of the bonuses or side effects is that the person will undergo this kind of awe-full moment.

One goal is to become the qualitatively whole new person you can become. Picture that you begin a session as the person you are, and then picture that by the end of the session you are a qualitatively whole new person. A transformation has happened. It may last only a few minutes or so, or it may last for a long time. You look qualitatively different. The feelings in you are qualitatively new. So is the way you think, act, and behave in your world. There is a basic, a fundamental, a deep-seated qualitative shift in who and what you are. You live and exist in a qualitatively new world. What is "out there" is as different and as new as the person you are inside. The change is awesome.

Nor do you undergo just any change. You become the person that you and you alone are capable of becoming. The chances are that you will ordinarily spend your entire life without undergoing a radically deep-seated change. The chances are that you have little or no idea of the person you are capable of being. As surprising and outlandish as it may seem, a goal of every experiential session is to enable you to undergo this incredible qualitative change into being the whole new person that you are capable of being. This goal sets the stage for your going through these kinds of awe-full moments.

The other goal is being free of the painful scene and feelings that were front and center for you in the session. By the end of the session, the related other goal is that the qualitatively whole new person no longer has the painful, hurtful, bad feelings in the painful, hurtful, bad scene that was so pronounced for the person you were when you began the session. The personal world in which you live is now essentially free of that painful situation and, if the situation is still roughly in your world, it is somehow different, less painful, less welded to painful feelings in you. You may start the session with a painful scene of being hated, rejected, shoved away by the one to whom you entrusted yourself. By the end of the session, your world no longer contains such scenes and such feelings in those scenes.

These are the goals of each experiential session. They are admittedly radical, powerful, ambitious.

These are the same goals of an experiential session with a teacher-therapist. When you have your own experiential session, you are the one who knows what to do and how to do it. You guide yourself through the session. You are the one who says or thinks, "Now I have to do this, and here is the way I do this," or you know all of this so well that you just do it without saying it out loud or even thinking it.

When you have a session with an experiential teacher, that part of what you do is handed to the experiential teacher. The teacher is the one who is responsible for telling you what to do and how to do it. You do the work. The teacher guides and steers you. The teacher is the one who says, "Now you are to do this, and here is the way you do this."

That is perhaps the main difference between having your own experiential session and having a session with an experiential teacher-therapist. The goals of the sessions are the same. What you accomplish ought to be the same whether you have your own experiential session or have a session with an experiential teacher-therapist.

THESE ARE THE STEPS YOU GO THROUGH IN ALMOST EVERY EXPERIENTIAL SESSION YOU HAVE BY YOURSELF

Each experiential session has a beginning, a middle, and an ending. Each session goes through the same steps as every other session. If you listen to a number of sessions carried out by the same person, it would likely seem that each is a session in and of itself, and it would be hard to tell if this was an earlier or a later session. Each session is to go through the same four steps:

Step 1. Discover the deeper potential for experiencing. The aim of the first step is to access, to bring forth, to find, to discover something that is deep down inside you. Picture this as a potentiality for some kind of experiencing, a deeper potential for experiencing that is typically outside your awareness. Start by putting yourself in a state of welcoming readiness for undergoing relatively strong feeling. Then find a scene of quite strong feeling, either good or bad feeling, from your current world or from long ago. Let yourself fully enter into, live and be in, this scene, and actively search for the exact instant of peak feeling. The deeper potential for experiencing can be discovered when you enter down inside that precious instant of peak feeling.

Step 2. Welcome, accept, cherish the deeper potential for experiencing. The purpose of the second step is to achieve a new state of genuinely loving, welcoming, embracing, cherishing what you had kept sealed off deep down inside, that discovered deeper potential for experiencing.

Step 3. Undergo a qualitative shift into being that deeper potential for experiencing in the context of earlier life scenes. The third step is achieved when you wholly disengage from, no longer are, the ordinary person you have been, and instead enter wholly and completely into being the utterly new person who is that formerly deeper potential for experiencing. This is accomplished by wholly living and being this qualitatively new person in the context of scenes from the past.

Step 4. Be the qualitatively whole new person in scenes from the forthcoming new post-session world. In the final step, the qualitatively whole new person has an ample sample and taste, readiness and commitment to live and be the whole new person in this new person's new world of today, tomorrow, and beyond. Step 4 provides for trying out, for sampling, for rehearsing, for shaping and refining, and then for actually experiencing what it is like to be the qualitatively new person in the qualitatively new post-session world.

In an experiential session, one moment of sheer awe occurs as you begin step 1, a second moment occurs in step 3, and the third occurs toward the end of step 4.

An experiential session with a teacher-therapist goes through the same steps in the same way. If you were to follow an experiential session carried out by a person alone and another session in which there is an experiential teacher-therapist present, the two sessions would follow the same steps and proceed through the session in much the same way. This ought not come as a surprise because the goals of both sessions are identical, and because most people who have sessions with an experiential teacher-therapist are geared toward learning how to eventually have their own sessions by themselves.

WHAT ARE THE THREE AWE-FULL MOMENTS IN YOUR EXPERIENTIAL SESSION?

The emphasis here is on your having your own experiential sessions. Yet it is almost certain that you will have the same three awe-full moments whether you go through the session by yourself or with an experiential teacher-therapist. What are these three awe-full moments?

1. The First Awe-Full Moment Is When You Say Yes, and Actually Throw Yourself into Having an Experiential Session That Can End the Very Existence of the Very Person You Are

The first awe-full moment is when you take the first step of committing yourself to going through a session that can alter the essential person you are. The moment is when you are in the room, your eyes are closed, and you commit yourself to carrying out the first step.

When you stand at the very edge, when you can either hurl yourself into a session or draw safely back, when you stand poised at the edge of the precipice, are you really ready to commit yourself, to submit yourself, to a session that can change you forever, that can put you through a wholesale qualitative, wrenching change into being the radically new person you can become, whatever that may be? You know that the two goals are wondrous, precious, all-powerful. Achieving them means a total commitment. The machinery is ready. Only you can turn it on. Once you say yes, once you turn it on, it stays on until the session has done its work, until the session is over. Take your time. The choice is yours.

Picture that you are in a room. You hear the voice of your therapist-teacher or, if you are alone, you hear the voice of the method. The voice says, "Are you truly ready to go through this session, never to turn back until the session is over, no matter what happens, no matter how long it takes? Are you truly ready to commit and dedicate yourself completely? If you are ready, say yes loud and clear. If you are ready, say YES . . . NOW!"

If you are, in this instant, fully committed to say yes, if you are wholly dedicated to say yes, then, if we freeze this tiny instant, there is almost always a fraction of a second of awe, of the ecstasy and terror of fully committing and submitting yourself to undergoing a session of absolute transformation, of undergoing the qualitative change into becoming a radically new person.

Most people never reach this moment. You spend your life staying safely away from this edge, and from the awe-full instant of committing yourself to hurling yourself over the edge and into a session of deepest change.

This is the first moment of sheer awe in a precious experiential session.

2. The Second Awe-Full Moment Is When You Say Yes, and Actually Throw Yourself into Fully and Completely Being the Qualitatively Whole New Person You Can Be

The second moment comes after you have discovered something deep inside you. It is a hidden deeper quality, a way of being, a possibility for a kind of experiencing, a deeper potentiality for experiencing. It is so deep inside that you have rarely if ever felt it, undergone it, even known that it was there. It is that deep inside you.

But now you do have a clear shot at what it is. You see it up close and in detail. You have discovered a deeply hidden, whole new way of being, a possibility or potentiality for experiencing. Suppose it is a deeper possibility for experiencing being in charge, in control, domination. This is not at all a part of the person you are. This is not part of your daily being or undergoing or feeling or experiencing. Once in a rare while, you may touch lightly on a tiny token sample, but this is not you, not a part of the person you are. It is sealed off, hidden, deep within you.

You also have found a scene, a situation in which you certainly were not this way. You were the way you usually were in that situation: kindly, understanding, gracious, compromising. The scene happened last night when the whole family was at your place, trying to decide what to do with poor old Momma, who is getting more and more gloomy since Daddy died last year. The whole family is politely skating around topics everyone is astutely complicit in not directly talking about. The scene was explicitly when you did your gracious best to head off the usual confrontation between your older brother and your nasty aunt.

The moment of awe comes when you go back into that scene, just before you actually launched into being the level-headed compromiser between your explosive older brother and your nasty aunt. If we freeze this instant, are you ready for an earth-shattering change, a massive transformation? Are you ready, instead of being the person you were, are you truly ready to undergo a truly catastrophic shift into being a qualitative, radical, wholesale new person who is not at all you, but is the living embodiment of being completely in charge, completely dominating, in absolute control? You are to undergo being this altogether new and different person fully, with supercharged gusto, in full force, all the way, with full vigor and intensity. Let yourself be this whole new person totally free of all reality constraints, in total silliness, zaniness, wildness, and with unbounded exhilaration and excitement.

All right. You are indeed living and being in the scene. It is that instant when Aunty has just said, "Sam ought to care for Mom. He's got all the money in the family!" and you see older brother Sam's lid about to explode. Right here, in this very frozen instant, are you absolutely ready to throw yourself into being this whole new other person who is the sheer experiencing of in charge, control, domination? Yes. Then throw yourself into being it . . . NOW!

If we freeze what happens, and if you have chosen to say yes, and if you have thrown yourself into being this whole new person in this real moment, then there is a fraction of an instant in which you have absolutely let go of every last shred of being the ordinary continuing you, you have passed the point of no return in becoming the qualitatively new person who is the pure experiencing of being in absolute change, complete control, full domination, and you have a flash of awe, of wonder and excitement, of fright and terror.

This is the second moment of awe in a precious session. It is the instant of having passed the point of no return in your letting go of the very person you have existed as, and into actually being the utterly new, radically new, qualitatively new person who is the deeper potential for experiencing that you had kept hidden and sealed off throughout your whole existence.

3. The Third Awe-Full Moment Is When You Say Yes, and You Continue Being the Qualitatively New Person in the Qualitatively New Post-Session World

Now you truly are a whole new person in this session. You have undergone the qualitative switch, the radical conversion, the dramatic transformation. For perhaps the first time in your life, almost certainly in your current life, there is a whole new part to the whole new you. It feels peaceful and exciting to have a sense of being in charge. It feels right and joyful to have a sense of absolute control. It feels natural and alive to have this wonderful sense of domination.

In the final part of the session, you were living and being this whole new person in all sorts of scenes and situations from the post-session world. You sampled what life can be like as this qualitatively new person who leaves the session and lives and exists in the imminent new world out there, in the whole new world of this whole new person. The new person had a foretaste, a preview, of what life can be like when the door opens and the new you walks into the world of today, tomorrow, and maybe forever.

You are being far more than just the formerly deeper potential for experiencing. You are far more than merely the new experiencing of being in charge, being in absolute control, of experiencing this newfelt domination. This formerly deeper potential is now an integral part of a whole new you. You have become a whole new person that includes this whole new, and integrated, potentiality for experiencing.

What is more, this whole new person lives in a whole new world that is essentially free of those old painful scenes and situations, and the whole new person is essentially free of the painful feelings in those painful situations.

As the session comes to an end, you are this qualitatively whole new person, and you are ready to end the session and to enter into a qualitatively whole new world that fits nicely with the qualitatively whole new person that you are.

Suppose that we freeze this moment, hold it still. In this very moment, you can remain being this whole new person, and when you open your eyes and walk out of the room, you can live and be in a new world out there. Or, in this precious moment, you can switch back into being the ordinary you that you have always been, the you whom you were in the beginning of the session.

This is the third awe-full moment in virtually every experiential session. Who is here? Who is this person whom you are? Are you the qualitatively new person who opens your eyes, walks out of the room, and lives in a new world? Being this new person is marvellously available. Or will you, in this frozen awe-full moment, revert back to the ordinary person you have almost always been?

In this frozen moment, there is an instant where the decision has to be made. You must choose, one way or the other. Which is it to be? The choice is here. You must choose yes to remain or you choose no and you revert back. And your choice is . . . !? Here is the moment of awe, filled with excitement and wonder, and with dread and fright. It all happens in a brief moment.

In this brief moment, perhaps we can appreciate how and why awe can include such a sense of ecstasy, wonder, fascination. Perhaps it comes from the incredible transformation, from having stepped into being the new person. Being this new person now, and being able to be this new person from now on, forever, can be awe-full. And when awe is accompanied with dread, terror, primal fear? Perhaps this third awe-full moment allows us to know how easy it is to step back into the ordinary you, how easy it is to see how we actually may choose to step back into a personal world of pain, suffering, hurt, anguish. We deliberately choose to return to this world of pain and terrible feelings. It is as if the dread, the terror, the primal fear are from having the choice of becoming and remaining the qualitatively whole new person or of watching our selves clinging to worlds of pain, suffering, hurt, anguish (cf. Binswanger, 1967; May, Angel, & Ellenberger, 1958).

THESE AWE-FULL MOMENTS COMMONLY OCCUR INSIDE OF AND UNCOMMONLY OCCUR OUTSIDE OF EXPERIENTIAL SESSIONS

The common notion of awe is large enough, flexible enough, and friendly enough to agree that, even though a sense of awe is rare and is to be treasured, it can happen under lots of circumstances, in lots of places. A person can undergo a sense of awe when seeing the birth of a baby, being in the presence of God, opening one's eyes and truly seeing radiant colors, watching the sun rise, being deeply understood by the other, being transfixed by the miraculous change, waking up to the utter beauty of fullsome nature, coming to the cataclysmic realization, being transfixed by the sheer power of a tornado or a full eclipse. However, there is a particular kind of awe-full moment that is a precious characteristic of experiential sessions.

THIS PARTICULAR KIND OF AWE-FULL MOMENT IS WHEN YOU HAVE PASSED THE POINT OF NO RETURN IN THE AWE-FULL FINAL LEAP

The particular kind of awe-full moment I am referring to is one that occurs when you have taken that momentous step into the complete and utter commitment of the final leap, when you have gone beyond the point of no return and you are in the throes of the final leap into the black abyss, into giving up everything of who and what you are, into a wholesale sacrificing of your entire self, into the bottomless pit of the unseeable unknown, into the cataclysmic ultimate change, into the final oblivion, into the final leap into the void of absolute death of oneself, into the existential meaning of suicide.

The stakes are almost as high as they can be. The risk is the ultimate risk of certain death, eternal nothingness, the end of your existence, or the risked possibility of the becoming of a whole new person, of absolute transformation, of qualitative metamorphosis, of an entirely new existence. This is the particular kind of awe-full moment that may perhaps rarely occur outside of experiential sessions, but is a precious characteristic of experiential sessions themselves.

What is so precious is the moment of being in the final leap, rather than the accompanying feeling of awe. From the experiential perspective (Mahrer, 1989, 1996), what is so precious, what is celebrated and valued, is having committed oneself to this final leap, the actual undergoing of this final leap, the being in it, the feeling and experiencing of it. Something is magnificently different in you in this moment. You are committed. You are in the actual throes of the final leap. You are no longer quite the person you had been just before. All of this is what is so precious, rather than the accompanying feeling or state of awe.

In this precious moment, there is no one to bathe in this accompanying sense of awe. You would have to stop, turn to the side, and expose yourself to the awe that is nearby. You are not undergoing this awe that is here. You are not facing what can inspire the sense of awe. In this moment, there is little or no appreciation of this sense of awe. The sense or feeling or state of awe is simply not important in this precious moment. The burst of awe in this awe-full moment is merely a wonderful automatic brief accompaniment of truly being in this final leap. It is an indication, a lovely momentary sign, of actually being in this final leap. You will pass by this puff of awe as you descend in the final leap. Yes, this is an awe-full moment. No, you are not filled with awe.

MOST PEOPLE RARELY KNOW THE PRECIOUS MOMENT OF HAVING COMMITTED ONESELF TO THE FINAL LEAP

Each experiential session offers you a golden opportunity to undergo the final leap of departing from, of letting go of, the whole person who you are, and falling headlong into the risked possibility of becoming the person you can become. In stark contrast, most people go through their entire lives without undergoing even a single moment of having committed oneself to that final leap. For almost every person, living from day to day, year after year, has few if any moments when the person actually commits oneself to giving up their very existence, sacrificing that everpresent sense of self, actively letting go of that sense of "I-ness," letting go of the precious core of who and what the person is, stepping away from the innermost spark of being oneself, resolutely ending the living center of one's actual existence.

This precious moment is not quite the same as drifting into death. This precious moment comes from actively placing oneself in the position of being ready to undertake the final leap, of then hurling oneself into that final leap, and of knowing the sense of having passed the point of no return. Most people have never known what this tiny moment is like.

THERE ARE PLENTY OF FEARS TO PROTECT YOU FROM ACTUALLY UNDERGOING THE AWE-FULL FINAL LEAP

You may come close to the edge. You may even lean perilously forward. But there are plenty of fears that can rescue you from the final leap.

There is a fear of losing control, of giving up that moment-by-moment control that is almost always there. There is a fear of becoming uncivilized, out of control, wild, animal-like. There is a fear of craziness, lunacy, derangement, losing your mind. There is a fear that inspires codes of ethics, morality, values, laws, familial and community and societal recrimination and punishment. There is a fear of the unknown, the empty blackness, the endless void. There is a fear of death, of the ending of your very existence. Before you commit yourself to the final leap, these fears snap into place and insure that you never undergo the awe-full final leap.

First there is the lure, the promise, the goal. Are you really passionate about undergoing wondrous change and becoming all that you can become? Are you passionate about being free of your hurts and pains, your personal anguishes and sufferings? If your ready answer is yes, then all you have to do is to undergo the awe-full final leap. Now come the fears. I must undergo that awe-full final leap? Yes. This is the requirement. It is as if you choose to keep all the hurts and pains, to remain the person with the anguishes and the sufferings, to decline undergoing the wondrous transformation into becoming all that you can become. You choose remaining in this state rather than succumbing to all the fears that protect you from actually undergoing the awe-full final leap. Isn't this interesting?

CONCLUSIONS AND INVITATION

1. There are particular kinds of awe-full moments that commonly occur in most experiential sessions and uncommonly occur outside of these sessions.
2. Experiential sessions can occur by and with oneself or with an experiential teacher-therapist.
3. If these particular kinds of awe-full moments appeal to you, the invitation is to learn how to have your own experiential sessions.
4. You are invited to read the following article for a first-hand account of one person's having their own experiential session and going through these particular kinds of awe-full moments.

REFERENCES

Binswanger, L. (1967). *Being-in-the-world.* New York: Harper.

Mahrer, A. R. (1989). *Experiencing: A humanistic theory of psychology and psychiatry.* Ottawa: University of Ottawa Press.

Mahrer, A. R. (1996). *The complete guide to experiential psychotherapy.* New York: John Wiley and Sons.

May, R., Angel, E., & Ellenberger H.F. (Eds.) (1958). *Existence: A new dimension in psychiatry and psychology.* New York: Basic Books.

What It Was Like
to Go Through Three Awe-Full Moments
in My Own Experiential Session

Anthony D. Firestone

SUMMARY. I am neither a psychotherapist nor a client. I am a person who is learning how to have his own experiential sessions. The purpose of this article is to describe a session with emphasis on three awe-filled moments that can occur in most experiential sessions. These three awe-filled moments were studied by means of in-depth examination of an audiotape of the session. *[Article copies available for a fee from The Haworth Document Delivery Service: 1-800-342-9678. E-mail address: <getinfo@haworthpressinc.com> Website: <http://www.HaworthPress.com> © 2001 by The Haworth Press, Inc. All rights reserved.]*

KEYWORDS. Awe-full moments, life scenes, choice, rehearsing, being passive

A LITTLE ABOUT ME AND MY EXPERIENTIAL SESSION

I have an upper management job in state government. Jean and I have been married for twenty years. We have two teen-aged daughters. Jean is a high

---

Address correspondence to: Anthony D. Firestone, c/o Alvin R. Mahrer, PhD, School of Psychology, University of Ottawa, Ottawa, Ontario, Canada K1N 6N5.

Author note: In my job, I write plenty of in-house reports, but never anything that was published. My wife, Jean, should be co-author because she showed me how to rewrite almost every sentence in draft after draft. I should also acknowledge Al Mahrer because he asked me to write this, he sent me a copy of the preceding article, and he was so helpful in organizing what I was trying to say, and what Jean showed me how to say.

[Haworth co-indexing entry note]: "What It Was Like to Go Through Three Awe-Full Moments in My Own Experiential Session." Firestone, Anthony D. Co-published simultaneously in *The Psychotherapy Patient* (The Haworth Press, Inc.) Vol. 11, No. 3/4, 2001, pp. 141-147; and: *Frightful Stages: From the Primitive to the Therapeutic* (ed: Robert B. Marchesani, and E. Mark Stern) The Haworth Press, Inc., 2001, pp. 141-147. Single or multiple copies of this article are available for a fee from The Haworth Document Delivery Service [1-800-342-9678, 9:00 a.m. - 5:00 p.m. (EST). E-mail address: getinfo@haworthpressinc.com].

school teacher, used to be a reporter, and she teaches writing skills. Neither of us have had anything to do with professional psychotherapists except that one of our friends is a student counselor at the high school where Jean teaches.

I can't think of some dramatic problem or big personal trouble. Lately I have been putting on too much weight, and I worry that my department might be swallowed up in a sweeping reorganization, but probably the biggest thing I worry about is that my father died about a year ago and I don't think my mother can live alone anymore.

My name is not Anthony D. Firestone. Jean and I knew I had to use a pseudonym even before the first draft was done. Whether we thought of our daughters, colleagues where I work or where Jean works, neighbors, friends of ours, anyone, the conclusion was the same: use a pseudonym.

Over a year ago, Jean and I went to an introductory workshop on having your own experiential sessions. We liked the idea, and went through a three-day training session so that we could have our own experiential sessions. Learning consisted of trying to have three or four sessions, with solid help from a teacher who listened to audiotapes of my sessions and gave me suggestions for how to do it better. Then I had the session I want to tell you about. It was awesome.

THE FIRST AWE-FULL MOMENT WAS WHEN I KNEW THIS SESSION COULD ACTUALLY BRING ABOUT A HUGE CHANGE IN ME AND MY LIFE

After this session, I knew that the three or four previous sessions were actually kind of light. Even as I started those sessions, I knew nothing dramatic would happen. I knew I would not risk anything serious, anything truly big and important in me or in my life.

Then something happened. Our older daughter is sixteen. She and a girlfriend were studying at the dining room table, books and notebooks all over. They both got up, I think to get something to drink from the kitchen. That was when I first saw that girl. I was stunned. It was like being hit by a thunder bolt. I was transfixed. I was struck dumb. And I stayed that way for four days!

The main thing is that I could not get that image of her out of my mind. It is hard to describe her and what exactly I felt. In a way, there was nothing conspicuously extraordinary about her. She seemed pretty, but not unusually so. She did not seem to ooze sex or be some angel or some demonic figure. But there was something about that young woman that was like a powerful magnet. I felt utterly compelled by her, drawn toward her, engrossed with her. I spent almost every minute of the next four days thinking of her, seeing mental images of her.

During those days, I did not do anything weird, risky, unusual, dangerous. I did not even think about doing anything like that. I did not secretly follow her around, ask my daughter about her friend, find out where she lived, paint pictures of her.

Nor did my life fall apart. I did not wander the streets at night, stop going to work, pick fights at work, lose my appetite, stare vacantly into space, stay up all night. I just kept seeing that girl in my mind's eye, almost constantly.

I think I was in such a state that I was just engrossed. I did not stop being engrossed with that image of that girl to have worries about what was happening to me. I was so busy being engrossed that I would not have been able to tell Jean what happened, or to talk it over, even a little bit, with my best friend, or to be worried about what was going on and what might happen.

Nevertheless, those were the most powerful and unusual days of my life. I think I know now that I was just a few inches away from me and my life falling apart. It would not have taken much for me to go out of my mind, to end up in court, to lose Jean and my daughters and my job. Thankfully, nothing happened.

After four days of this, I had an experiential session. I walked into the room, shut the door, turned on the tape recorder, leaned back in the recliner, and closed my eyes. I was ready to begin. For a few seconds I was quiet, and then the first awe-full moment happened.

The whole meaning of a session changed. Suddenly, an experiential session had power, awesome power. I knew I would get to the bottom of this craziness with this girl. I knew that I would be different in some big way. I knew that my life would be altogether different somehow. This session could really change me. Well? Am I ready to have a session? It felt like everything inside me said yes. That was when I felt the first awe-full moment. I had put myself into the hands of a session that could change everything and, in the awe-full moment, I flipped the switch to begin. The awe-full moment was in the instant after flipping the switch. The show was on!

THE SECOND AWE-FULL MOMENT WAS IN THE FRACTION OF A SECOND WHEN I THREW MYSELF INTO BEING THE WHOLE NEW PERSON, AND PASSED THE POINT OF NO RETURN

An experiential session starts when you find a scene that is filled with powerful feeling. I certainly had my scene. It was when I first saw that girl as she stood up from her chair in the dining room.

Once you find a scene of strong feeling, there are procedures to help you probe inside the scene, to go deep inside yourself, and to find out what is there deep inside you. Starting from that scene, I found something so surprising, so far beyond anything I remember feeling any time in my life. I discovered that deep inside me was the possibility of experiencing a sense of being utterly taken over, completely passive, fully giving in. It was more than something sexual. It seemed completely new to me. Al Mahrer calls it a deeper potential for experiencing. I think of it as a whole different person hidden somewhere deep inside me.

Once you discover a deeper possibility for experiencing in you, there are methods to help you to accept it, even to feel good about it. I did this.

Then comes the dramatic step. It starts by finding scenes from the past. I came up with a scene from when I was seven years old. My mother used to drive me to hockey practice on Saturday mornings. Very early on Saturday mornings. I hated hockey. Mom and Dad loved hockey. I am supposed to be eating my cereal. I am not eating this lumpy hot cereal. I am grumpy and whining about being tired. Mom is across the table, dressed and ready to get in the car, and giving me looks of how disgusting I am.

According to the method, I am supposed to actually be in this scene as if I am really being the seven-year-old not eating the hot lumpy cereal. Then, and here is the dramatic part, I am literally to switch over into being a whole new kid who is the pure experiencing of being utterly taken over, completely passive, fully giving in. I am gone, and in my place is this whole other kid who doesn't even sound like me. He is a whole new person who thinks, acts, talks, and is the whole new person. It is to be a dramatic change.

When I listened to the tape, the dramatic switch from being the seven-year-old me to being that whole new kid happened in about a second. I tried to hold that second still, to keep it here, to dilate it, and to dissect what I think happened in that crucial second.

I remembered, in the session, having a brief flash of what that other little boy might be like. I could see what it could be like to be a whole different kid, sitting there, and thoroughly enjoying being utterly taken over by Mother's wanting him to be good, being completely passive to Mother's hopes and wishes for him, fully giving in to Mother's understandable dismay at his reluctant slowness.

In that dilated moment, I remember actually deciding to go ahead and to hurl myself into being this whole other little boy. And then I thought I remembered falling into, and being swallowed into, being this whole new person. I think it was just around this frozen instant when I had a flash of sadness or loss that I was no longer me, and fear that it was too late, the die was cast. I think I also had a flash of excitement, of thrill, that I was about to be a whole new person.

When I read Al Mahrer's article, and when I listened so carefully to that moment in the audiotape, I think that was a moment of awe. However, during the actual session, I had no sense of this at all. That switch happened much too quickly, and I was much too busy actually going through the radical change of becoming the whole new person in that childhood scene in the kitchen.

THE FINAL AWE-FULL MOMENT WAS JUST BEFORE THE SESSION ENDED, AND I WOKE UP TO BEING ME AGAIN, NO LONGER THE WHOLE NEW PERSON I HAD BECOME

Once the incredible switch happened, once I actually became the new person, I stayed being this new person throughout the session, or almost. It was actually easy, and great fun, to find scene after scene from my past, and to be this new person who revels in the experiencing of being utterly taken over, completely passive, fully giving in. It felt wonderful, so alive, and so natural. I really was a substantially new person in scene after scene.

In the final step of the session, I was to continue being this new person, but I was to move from past scenes to scenes from the next few days or so. The method has me forget about reality constraints, what would really happen if I were actually like this. Instead, I was to pump up the sheer silliness and giddiness of being this whole new person in forthcoming scenes that were to be unrealistic, make-believe, like a cartoon or wacky comedy, with plenty of energy and gusto and fun.

I had a festival of being this new person in all sorts of imminent scenes, even in scenes involving that girlfriend of my daughter's.

The session is to end with my still being this whole new person, except that the context is now to be much more realistic. As this new person, when and where do I really want to be this person in the real world after the session?

I knew that I am to find or to create some scenes, to turn on the bright lights of reality constraints, to see what it can be like to be this whole new person in this whole new real world, to choose at least one scene, to rehearse it, to give all parts of me plenty of opportunity to voice their objections, and then to decide if I am really ready to commit myself to being this whole new person in that new scene in the new real world.

I found a place. Each week I have a meeting with the heads of the departments I administer. With the reality lights turned on, I actually reveled in rehearsing what it could be like to be this whole new person in the meeting, doing all sorts of things that gave me a wonderful sense of being utterly taken over, completely passive, fully giving in.

That was when the third awe-full moment happened. In this moment, I could remain being the new person or I could switch back. Suddenly I was no longer this whole new person. Instead, it was like "I" woke up. I was once again the person I had been. I had switched back to being me, no longer this new person.

When I think about that moment now, watch it in very slow motion, and see what happened during that moment, I remember a split second when I, as this new person, seemed to halt, freeze. It was as if a decision was being made: Should I really be this whole new person from now on, or should I go back to being the person I was before the radical switch? I am serious about saying "a decision was being made" because it did not seem that "I" was making the decision, either as the whole new person or as the former old person. It seems eerie. I do remember, although I am not absolutely sure, that I felt a flash of fear about actually being this whole new person, and a flash of sadness at returning to being me again. The feeling was awe-full, but only for a split second.

WERE THERE ANY CHANGES AFTER THE SESSION?

One thing did not happen. I was not this whole new person in the meeting with my department heads. The meeting was fine. Most of them are, but no such new experiencing.

However, there was a dramatic change in my craziness about my daughter's girlfriend. It was gone! Somehow I got over those four days of being, I guess, out of my mind. What a relief. After my experiential session, when I saw her being with my daughter, I was still struck by something special about her, but things were different. I could appreciate that quality about her. She seemed like a real person with such a special quality. But now I felt solid, good, more like a real person.

One more thing, or lots of little things. In little unplanned ways, I started having mild new feelings of letting myself be taken over, being passive, giving in. The first time was a few days after the session when Jean and I were cross-country skiing. I started falling into the rhythm of the swish of the skis, and giving in to the sight of the glistening snow on the trail, and the feel of the sun on my face, the pleasant enjoyment of the tingling in my muscles. Jean mentioned the self-satisfied new little grin all across my face as we were skiing. This new experiencing also made subtly nice new differences when Jean and I made love, when I started lingering longer in showers, when I drifted into falling asleep when I went to bed, and when Jean and I had pleasant interludes of easy talking about whatever we found ourselves talking about.

I AM PROUD OF GOING THROUGH THE THREE AWE-FULL MOMENTS

Maybe "proud" isn't quite the right word, but it comes close. Going through those three awe-full moments seems so important. I think I am proud of actually submitting myself to something that can actually wrench me into becoming a new person. It is exciting to take the leap. I know how easy it can be to just coast through life without ever even facing the risk of such a leap.

I think I am proud of throwing myself into actually being that whole new person in scenes from the past. It was exhilarating, exciting, inspiring, awesome to enter into being a whole new person, from top to bottom, from inside out. I have no memory of actually going through this at any time in my life until now.

When I was this new person in the session, I faced a powerful choice of being this whole new person in the real world, after the session, or going back to being the person I had seen. I am proud that I put myself into the position of facing this awesome choice. In a way, being in a position of facing this choice was more important than whatever choice I made.

Now that I have tried to describe what it was like to have gone through the three awe-full moments in the session, I suspect it might be easier for me to go through my experiential sessions.

The Role of Awe in Experiential Personal Construct Psychology

L. M. Leitner

SUMMARY. This article begins by elaborating an experiential personal construct psychology definition of reverence. A discussion of the experience of reverence in the therapy relationship begins by focusing on
the therapist's reverence of the client and is followed by an exploration
of the therapist accepting the client's reverence. Ways that the therapist
and client can retreat from the experience of the reverential also are explored. Finally, I discuss the experience of transpersonal reverence
within experiential personal constructivism. *[Article copies available for a
fee from The Haworth Document Delivery Service: 1-800-342-9678. E-mail
address: <getinfo@haworthpressinc.com> Website: <http://www.HaworthPress.
com> © 2001 by The Haworth Press, Inc. All rights reserved.]*

KEYWORDS. Relationships, contact, emptiness, meaningfulness, resistances, distress, transference, reverence, validation, intimacy, anger, sexuality,
fear

L. M. Leitner, PhD, is Professor of Psychology at Miami University. He has
published over 50 books, chapters, and articles dealing with various topics relevant to
humanistic psychology. He is on the Editorial Board for the *Journal of Constructivist
Psychology* and *The Psychotherapy Patient*. He is a Fellow of the American Psychological Association and President-Elect of APA's Division of Humanistic Psychology.

Address correspondence to: L. M. Leitner, PhD, Department of Psychology,
Miami University, Oxford, OH 45056 USA (E-mail: LEITNELM@muohio.edu).

Author note: I would like to thank Linda Endres, Lara Honos-Webb, Derek
Oliver, and especially April Faidley for comments on an earlier version of this paper.
All clinical material has been distorted to protect confidentiality.

Based upon a paper presented at the annual meeting of the American Psychological Association, Boston, MA, August, 1999.

[Haworth co-indexing entry note]: "The Role of Awe in Experiential Personal Construct Psychology."
Leitner, L. M. Co-published simultaneously in *The Psychotherapy Patient* (The Haworth Press, Inc.) Vol. 11,
No. 3/4, 2001, pp. 149-162; and: *Frightful Stages: From the Primitive to the Therapeutic* (ed: Robert B.
Marchesani, and E. Mark Stern) The Haworth Press, Inc., 2001, pp. 149-162. Single or multiple copies of this
article are available for a fee from The Haworth Document Delivery Service [1-800-342-9678, 9:00 a.m. - 5:00
p.m. (EST). E-mail address: getinfo@haworthpressinc.com].

Experiential personal construct psychology (Leitner, 1988) is an approach to understanding persons in the light of their struggles in interpersonal relationships: the desire for relational depth versus needing to limit it. Based upon George Kelly's (1991a, 1991b) Sociality Corollary, experiential personal construct psychology assumes that deeply significant interpersonal contact (termed "ROLE relationships" in the theory) is essential to a life of richness and meaning. On the other hand, such relationships can be filled with fear, as they are the very relationships that can be the most damaging in life. Thus, all persons confront the challenge of opening the self to an other, with the richness, meaning, and potential terror inherent in a ROLE relationship, or limiting the depth of relationships and paying the price of emptiness, meaninglessness, and guilt for the safety and protection that affords (see Leitner, 1985; Leitner & Faidley, 1995).

Experiential personal construct psychology has been elaborated into several areas of psychopathology and psychotherapy. These include a non-DSM approach to diagnosing human distress (Leitner, Faidley, & Celentana, 2000), an approach to assessment that combines experiential relevance with treatment implications (Leitner, 1995a; Faidley & Leitner, 1993), and an understanding of the optimally helpful therapy relationship (Leitner, 1995b). Focusing specifically on psychotherapy, the theory has been used to understand the ways clients validate and invalidate therapist interventions (Leitner & Guthrie, 1993), reasons for client resistances (Leitner & Dill-Standiford, 1993), the treatment of serious disturbances (Leitner & Celentana, 1997), differing bases for construing and misconstruing material as "unconscious" (Leitner, 1999), transference and countertransference (Leitner, 1997), and the need for therapist creativity in psychotherapy (Leitner & Faidley, 1999).

Experiential personal construct psychology also has considered the experience of the reverential. Leitner and Pfenninger (1994) described reverence as one of nine characteristics of optimal functioning. They defined reverence as "the awareness that one is validating the core ROLE process of the other" (p. 133). Putting this in less technical terms, reverence is experienced when I am aware that I am affirming your most central processes of being. Or, to put it even more experientially near, reverence is experienced when I am aware that I am in the presence of your "soul." Leitner and Faidley (1995) extended this initial discussion of reverence from an experiential personal construct perspective by elaborating the ways that ROLE relationships are "awful" and "aweful." Leitner (in press) further examined the ways that awe is experienced when the numbness associated with retreating from human intimacy has lifted in life-changing psychotherapy.

In this paper, I will begin with the technical definition of reverence and elaborate it to reflect the felt experience of reverence. The heart of the paper describes the therapeutic nature of both the therapist's and client's experience of reverence in therapy. Two aspects of interpersonal reverence are vital to this discussion: reverence for an other and the awareness that an other is revering you. In addition, the discussion would not be complete without dealing with the ways that the threat of reverence leads persons to withdraw from the experience. In a brief movement beyond the two types of reverence mentioned above, I will consider the role of a type of transpersonal reverence, the broadly experienced reverence for humanity.

REVERENCE DEFINED

As mentioned earlier, Leitner and Pfenninger defined reverence in terms of the awareness that one is validating the core ROLE processes of an other. Understanding this definition means understanding the technical terms of "validation," "core ROLE," and "process." In contrast to how personal construct psychology is commonly perceived, it is not a theory primarily concerned with "constructs" or meanings. Rather, it is much more concerned with our very process as meaning making creatures. It is the process of meaning creation and re-creation, more than any specific meanings, that is central to Kelly's theory (Leitner, 1985), as a perusal of his fundamental postulate and corollaries will demonstrate.

Process. Kelly's focus on process provides a powerful foundation for understanding interpersonal relations. "Kelly has made a distinction between construing things as the other person does and construing the other person's *process* of construing. It is like the distinction between seeing eye to eye with another and seeing from where the other is standing" (Faidley, 1993, pp. 13-14). If I focus on the content of your constructs, I may know that you size up the world in terms of "fairness versus unfairness," for example. While useful, this pales in understanding your process of construing. Understanding your process of meaning making gets me to your hopes, your dreams, your greatest fears, the ways you have been betrayed by others, your courage, your lack of courage, and so on. In the context of this knowledge of your process, your tendency to size up the world in terms of "fairness" can be understood much more richly and deeply. It is at this deeper, more significant, level of the process of your living that experiential personal construct psychology is most profoundly concerned.

Core ROLE. Our understandings of ourselves with regard to certain other people are central to life itself. These relational understandings of self and other are so deep and so vital that we often will act as if our very lives depend upon them (Kelly, 1991a). (Landfield, 1976, provided some empirical support for Kelly's position.) These central relational understandings are our core ROLE constructs. History is replete with examples of people choosing death over abandoning these core values, as, absent these central definers for the person, life was not worth living. These are the aspects of self that we risk in the meaningful, exciting, richly rewarding, terribly threatening world of ROLE relationships. In other words, in a reverential relationship, we hold the life-soul of the other in our hands.

Validation. Each time we act in the world, we are risking the affirmation or the disconfirmation of personal meanings. When I risk my heart and open myself deeply to you, you may invalidate me in innumerable ways. For example, you may use me as an object for your personal pleasure or further ego gratification. You may tell me that you are trustworthy and then betray me. You may change your mind and no longer desire any relational depth with me. When I am disconfirmed in such a way in a ROLE relationship, who I am as a person has been invalidated. After all, this disconfirmation attacks central definers of my process of living. Thus, ROLE relationships are filled with the potential for terror, even when we are not aware of it.

On the other hand, you may confirm (or validate) my decision to open myself deeply to you by how you respond to me. You may respect me, be kind to me, support me. However, you can go beyond this level of validation. You may hold my heart in your hand and respect it like the precious thing it is. You may treat my soul gently, as you know how fragile it can be. You may look at my personhood in all its nakedness and shame and see the decency behind it. When you are *aware* that you are holding my heart respectfully, treating my soul gently, and seeing the decency behind my shame and my retreats from others, you are revering me. I hope this all-too-brief discussion shows the ways that our technical definition attempts to honor the experience of reverence.

THERAPIST EXPERIENCE OF REVERENCE

The therapist's experience of reverence for the client can be transformative in the healing relationship of psychotherapy (Leitner & Faidley, 1995). Implicit in the definition of reverence is the fact that awe is experienced in a highly intimate relationship between two people. Thus, in any reverential experience, there is the integration of profound intimacy with a sense of separateness. This section will clarify how the therapist's ability to hold and balance closeness and distinctness promotes life-changing experiences in psychotherapy.

The credulous approach plus a professional understanding of distress. One aspect of good psychotherapy from an experiential personal construct perspective is the therapist's ability to simultaneously hold the profound connection and the separateness in her awareness. In this regard, Leitner and Faidley (1999) have argued that the therapist must simultaneously integrate a *credulous approach* (Kelly, 1991a) with a psychological understanding of the client's distress. The credulous approach is a way of understanding the client that mandates assuming that literally everything a client says is "true." Epting and Viney (1999), in describing the credulous approach, cite a case in which Carl Jung said that if a client told him that she had gone to the moon, she *really* went to the moon. Rather than trying to contradict the client, the therapist chooses to believe in the felt reality of the client's experience. In other words, we approach the client as if every communication reveals an important "truth" about the client.

In addition to experiencing the "truth" of the client's meaning system, the therapist must have ways of understanding human distress that offer the client opportunities for freedom and growth. Without this professional understanding, the only "reality" present in the therapy room is the client's. On the other hand, without the credulous approach, the only "reality" present in the therapy room is the therapist's. If either "reality" predominates, the therapeutic ROLE relationship is distorted and life-changing psychotherapy cannot occur. (Others also have said these two viewpoints are equally important in psychotherapy. Chessick, 1974, writing from a psychodynamic perspective, argued that the therapist needs to listen simultaneously from the world of the humanistic imagination and from the world of scientific understanding. His world of scientific understanding was a psychoanalytic understanding that allowed him to intervene around client resistances, transference distortions, and so on.)

For example, Faidley and Leitner (in press) describe Gena, who entered therapy after a near-lethal suicide attempt following the break up of her marriage. She reported a stormy childhood, filled with physical abuse and abandonment. Gena was extremely despairing over the divorce because it demonstrated that she did not "matter." Her therapist, rather than developing a professional understanding of "mattering," discussed how one can matter to someone who then changes his mind and that she could matter to friends, her children, and others. In response to these interventions, Gena became increasingly agitated and disorganized. Before the next appointment, she told people about reporting hearing voices telling her that she was Satan and she could matter to no one. The therapist, panicking, referred her to a psychiatrist for chemical control of her experience.

However, a friend talked Gena into seeing another therapist. This therapist understood "mattering" in a more symbolic way. He understood "mattering" as her yearning for that special relationship that young children deserve. A parent would never leave a child who "matters" to her parents as leaving one's child would be tantamount to leaving oneself. Gena responded dramatically to this interpretation. She cancelled her appointment with the psychiatrist as the hallucinations had ceased and she felt greater hope of being understood by her new therapist. In addition to credulously experiencing the panic behind not "mattering," this therapist also had a professional understanding of Gena's distress that helped her to grow beyond her current experience.

Optimal therapeutic distance. Optimal therapeutic distance (Leitner, 1995) is an experiential blending of connection with and separateness from the client. When I am optimally distant, I am near enough to my client's experience to feel it inside of me. At the same time, I am distant enough from my client's experience to recognize it as my client's, not my own. For example, consider Judy, a young woman who had been diagnosed as "psychotically depressed" by previous therapists. She reported a history of abuse that could best be summarized as torture. However, she also recalled pleasant times when her mother gave her bubble baths. During one discussion of these baths, she became horrified. She had remembered that, after the bubble baths, she was dressed in a nightgown and sexually abused by her stepfather. At this moment, I became aware of feeling a combination of sadness, shock, pain, outrage, and (unexpectedly) guilt. My emotional reactions permeated my interventions. For example, when she asked "Why did this happen?" I replied, with tenderness, "You blame yourself for it, don't you?" After sobbing for 10 minutes, Judy started talking about how she had always felt as if it were her fault because, if she could have been "good enough," they would not have treated her so horrifically. I would argue that the guilt I felt was my therapeutically experiencing Judy's emotion.

Both of these professional stances, the credulous approach and optimal therapeutic distance, reveal reverence for the client. In each of them, the therapist is aware of validating the core ROLE processes of the other. In so doing, the therapist provides the client with the most powerful human experience imaginable: the client can feel understood and respected down to his very soul. How can such an experience not transform both self and other?

THE THERAPIST'S RETREATS FROM REVERENCE

Despite the obvious power of therapeutic reverence, all too often therapists limit the depth of their engagement in therapy. Much of the time, this limiting is based upon the therapist's personal fears and past experiences. In this section of the paper, I will discuss some of the issues that limit the therapist's experience of reverence and, subsequently, the ability of the healing relationship to transform a life.

DSM diagnoses. The experiential personal construct definition of reverence explicitly describes viewing the other as a process of meaning creation and re-creation. This view of humans contrasts markedly with the current psychiatric nomenclature. The DSM-IV, like its predecessors, views people as a list of behaviors or a collection of static and disparaging traits. Rather than providing the clinician with a conceptual structure for grasping the subjective magnificence of the other, a DSM-influenced conceptualization makes the other into a non-human, a thing. This objectification (Honos-Webb & Leitner, in press) is extremely destructive to the subjective meaning making so central in the person-to-person connection of a ROLE relationship.

Honos-Webb and Leitner (in press) have described in detail the numerous ways a DSM-influenced conceptualization destroyed self-meanings for a young man being seen in therapy. Mike had no faith in his experiences and perceptions as he had been told he was "mentally ill" from early in his life. He also had no hope that a ROLE relationship might help him recover from relational injuries, since being "crazy" was viewed by mental health professionals as permanent. Jay Haley (see Farber, 1993) has stated that he gave up using terms like "schizophrenia" because professionals automatically assumed that such a "thing" was incurable.

Even if you were to argue that the DSM does not describe static entities, any perusal of the nomenclature comes up with demeaning description after demeaning description of persons in distress. There is no presentation of areas of strength, perseverance, insight, sensitivity, courage, or creativity. Should you doubt that, suppose I arranged a blind date with someone for you and the only thing you knew about this person was that she or he had a list of characteristics of a DSM diagnosis. Would you really be interested in going on this date?

In contrast to the DSM-like objectification, experiential personal constructivism focuses on what Kelly (1991b) called "transitive diagnosis." Transitive diagnosis involves arriving at a clinical understanding of the client that opens up possibilities for helping the client reinvent a meaningful life. Leitner, Faidley, and Celentana (2000) have described a way of understanding human meaning making that, we feel, meets Kelly's criteria for transitive diagnosis. The system combines a respect for the client's lived experience with potential pathways for helping the client transcend debilitating psychological injuries.

Rationing care. The profession seems to have accepted the current political view that "treatment" must be symptom-focused, short-term, and manualized. (See Bohart, O'Hara, & Leitner, 1998, for a critique of this position.) Forms from rationed-care companies (Miller, 1996) force clinicians to describe clients in terms of clusters of behaviors, self-defeating thoughts, genetic screw-ups, and/or biochemical phrenology. Therapists who feel they have to "play the game" with the care rationers are then forced into the terrible position of trying to simultaneously think one way in therapy with the client while speaking or writing another way when communicating with those who control reimbursement for services rendered. Laing (1969) called the belief that this is possible a self-delusion. Therapists who do not "play the game" face the economic insecurity of the possibility they may not get referrals from the care-rationing company. In either case, the therapist's concern with other issues limits the ability to engage the client in a transformative relationship.

The therapist's needs for professional respect. Therapists, like their clients, need the respect of their peers and colleagues. In this regard, the current socio-political climate of the profession is one that makes it all but impossible to revere clients while maintaining such respect. Caplan (1995) as well as Kutchins and Kirk (1997) have detailed the ways that the profession rewards people who think about clients in objectifying ways. Jim Mancuso (in Farber, 1993), a long-time critic of the DSM, has painted a picture of a young person entering graduate school with the hope of a career as a professor at a major university. She needs publications in mainline journals, references from people who do mainline psychology, etc. The odds of her choosing to work with people who are challenging the very system that will reward her handsomely are very small. In other words, to become the professional she hopes to be, she has to buy into the assumptions behind a medical model of psychopathology. She also has to buy into traditional research designs and statistics. Therefore, by the time she enters into the professional world, she has been socialized to think about humans in ways that make it difficult to revere the person seeking assistance.

The therapist's fears of intimacy. Therapists, like their clients, also have been injured in deeply personal relationships and have fears of relational contact. These fears of the person-to-person intimacy often manifest themselves in the therapist retreating from the client to a place of mutual, albeit superficial, comfort. For example, John was referred by his physician when he had sought help for his "flesh rotting away." In order to be helpful to John, I had to be able to emotionally resonate with the experience of being so disgustingly evil that you were rotten to the core. I could only do that by tapping into the parts of me that feel like I have been that evil at times (Leitner & Celentana, 1997). In other words, intimacy with John implied being in touch with parts of myself that I find disgusting, repugnant. How many times do therapists, when faced with this existential choice, choose to retreat behind toxic chemicals, concrete problem solving, or rational "reality testing"? How terrifying it is to say, with the emotional congruence that conveys beyond doubt that you *feel* what you are saying, "I know what it's like to feel so rotten that you think you are physically rotting away. I will be with you in that feeling and, in time, we will get beyond that."

The therapist's fears of anger. Deep relational contact exposes the therapist to intense emotions of many types. One that often is problematic to therapists is the client's rage. When confronted with fury, it is easy to withdraw into techniques, as opposed to continuing to connect with and hold onto the other. Therapist struggles with client anger can be particularly problematic when the fury is directed at the therapist. For example, soon after beginning to see me, John developed the delusion that the KGB was going to kill me. It would be easy to dismiss this experience as another manifestation of his "illness," to be dealt with through neurotoxins. However, respecting my client's experience means taking that experience seriously. I wondered what I had done that made him want to kill me. He replied that it was the KGB, not him, that wanted to kill me. I then talked about how, although it might be the KGB, I still wondered if it was some part of John. I said that I knew what it was like to want to kill someone. I also knew that we feel that way when we have been very badly hurt. I hoped that someday he could tell me how I had hurt him so that I would not do it again. After numerous sessions around this topic, the delusion disappeared. (As we will see below, there were other reasons for the delusion.)

The therapist's fears of sexuality. Intense contact also can result in sexual feelings that are frightening to the therapist. Susan sought therapy because of chronic depression and emptiness. It soon became apparent that she had lived a life with no intimate relationships at all, molding herself into whatever anyone wanted her to be. As she felt connected to me, she reported a dream of us having sex that was so intense that she awoke having an orgasm (Leitner, 1997). Rather than retreating from her due to my own fears about "inappropriately condoning a transference," I was able to share my sense that the dream suggested a freeing of emotional availability as well as reflecting her feeling increasingly connected to me.

As another example, John became quite upset and agitated a few months after the KGB delusion disappeared. He could not tell me what was happening other than making veiled references to men being interested in him sexually. Exploring this proved very difficult as John continued to see the problem as "their" being sexually interested in him. In a previous therapy, the therapist had prematurely interpreted this experience as John projecting his own homosexual impulses onto others, including the therapist. John became quite suspicious each time I said or did anything that might imply I thought he was projecting his homosexuality. The impasse finally broke when I was able to say, with feeling, to John, "Look. I do not know if you are gay or not. If you are, that's OK. If you're not, that's OK. What I do know is that sometimes when we have been badly hurt, we withdraw from people almost completely. When we start to find the courage within ourselves to care for others again, we sometimes confuse this caring with sex." This intervention allowed John to consider possibilities for his experience other than that he was sexually attracted to men. The reduced threat dissipated his fear of being judged and allowed him to bring his sexuality into therapy as a question to explore.

CLIENTS AND REVERENCE

Clients also can retreat from relational contact due to their fears of intimacy. Experiential personal constructivism argues that psychopathology can be understood as the retreating from ROLE relationships (due to the relational injuries we have sustained) and the consequent numbing of experience. Clients, according to this framework, are constantly simultaneously seeking out and protecting themselves from ROLE relationships. In this regard, they retreat from the experience of reverence in many of the same ways therapists retreat. However, in addition to these fears of revering the other, many seriously disturbed clients have a fear of being revered by an other, including the therapist.

Fear of being revered. Jim was in therapy after having had a panic attack when he started dating Betty. As we explored his experience of Betty, it became clear that he cared for her very deeply and respected her tremendously. He was quite frightened that Betty would see him for what he was and that he would not "measure up" in her eyes. I encouraged him to have a conversation with Betty about how she would describe him to her friends. Jim was upset the next session. He had asked Betty about this and she began describing his decency, honesty, caring, sensitivity, etc. Without being aware of what he was doing, Jim had curled into a ball and said, "That's enough" to Betty. As we explored why he was so threatened by her positive views of him, he was able to describe the terror he would feel if he were to trust Betty's view of him instead of his father's. Jim had never been a "real man" in his father's eyes. Believing that people could see him as an exceptional person in some ways meant believing that his father, rather than being the powerful protector, had been a source of injury. The parts of Jim that were still small, vulnerable, and needing a strong father could not tolerate the possibility that Betty was right.

As a final example, let us return to John and the KGB agents. This experience occurred shortly after we had made some progress on his flesh rotting away. As we stayed in the KGB area, what eventually became clear was that John was very frightened of the hope that was developing based upon our interactions. He had hoped innumerable times in the past only to have the "fabric of my soul" ripped apart. Being angry with me then accomplished many goals for John. First, it reflected his rage at my having done some things to hurt him. Second, it provided a screen to retreat behind and protect him from the possibility of being devastated again. Finally, it allowed him to experience how I would deal with his anger and his retreat. He then could use that knowledge to make a more informed decision about risking a ROLE relationship with me. All of this was beautifully and creatively encapsulated within the KGB delusion.

Experiencing reverence. As mentioned above, when clients can experience therapist reverence, powerful issues arise. The client can contrast this experience with the horrendous violence (both obvious and subtle–Leitner & Faidley, 1995) done to her in the past. She can contrast the deep experience of being valued and beautiful in the eyes of someone who knows her better than most people, to the experience of being ugly and despicable in the eyes of people who should have known her. Because contrast is inherent in meaning making (Kelly, 1991a; Rychlak, 1994), experiencing therapist reverence often leads to anger and anguish with regard to the injuries from our past.

Experiential personal constructivism assumes that we are inherently meaning making creatures. All experiences, then, are used by the client to re-create the meanings that form the bases of existence. Each experience of therapist reverence allows the self to be seen as a bit more worthwhile than previously thought possible. Further, as we re-create our very soul through these interactions, we eventually find that we no longer need retreats from intimacy that produce emptiness. Since we are relationship seeking, we may then choose to forgive those who have injured us in the past. (Leitner & Pfenninger, 1994, define forgiveness as reconstruing self and other such that past injuries do not prevent us from forming ROLE relationships in the future. Time does not allow me to explain how this technical definition can be seen experientially as forgiveness.) In so doing, we become free to *be*, perhaps for the first time in our lives.

Revering the other. Most ROLE relationships imply reciprocity (Leitner, 1985). In this regard, the experience of reverence in a ROLE relationship is not a one-way street. If we have a ROLE relationship, not only am I revering you; you are revering me. In this regard, many ROLE relationships are limited and made less powerful by denying the other the experience of revering me. Allowing the other in an intimate relationship to revere me can be seen as a *gift* that I give the other, as well as a gift that the other gives me (Leitner & Faidley, 1995). Depriving the other of this experience is damaging to self and other.

This issue can be quite confusing to therapists. Too often our discomfort with others' reverence of us results in our hurting our clients. We become concerned abut the "appropriateness" of the reverence. We become concerned about the ways the client's reverence (often manifesting itself in the form of profound gratitude) may be an "idealization." When we focus excessively on such concerns, we deny the client the experience of having his gift of reverence joyously accepted by an other. This can be a factor in undermining the sense of self we are co-creating with our client. People, whether clients or not, feel injured and betrayed when their experience of another is discounted as pathology. If we can overcome our own discomfort with being revered by an other, we can find ways of spontaneously accepting the reverence and exploring what other meanings it might have for the client.

Based upon the therapeutic relationship, the client will venture into the world of revering the other. In so doing, the client experiences the ways that giving and receiving are intricately intertwined in a ROLE relationship and it becomes difficult, if not impossible, to discuss any act as one person giving to (or receiving from) the other. The wonders of self and other can be mutually explored as the relationship develops and each person becomes more than they were before.

TRANSPERSONAL REVERENCE

Finally, I would like to briefly mention a specific form of reverence that goes beyond the I-Thou (Buber, 1970) reverence of a ROLE relationship. This is a reverence for all persons, based upon our shared humanity. Leitner and Faidley (1995) argued that this transpersonal reverence arises out of the interpersonal reverence discussed above. While people may do deeds for others that are quite helpful to the human condition, they are not necessarily based upon the revering of others. When transpersonal reverence is experienced, we become aware of the ways that limiting or depriving any person is an injury to the other, ourselves, and the entire human race.

Transpersonal reverence may develop out of repeated experiences of interpersonal reverence. We experience again and again the ways that such a relationship can transform self and other. As meaning making beings, we begin to see the ways that objectifying others injures and limits all of us. Just as we cannot meaningfully distinguish between the giver and the receiver in ROLE relationships as my receiving your gift is a gift to you and vice versa, so my objectification of you is an injury to me. As our clients develop a sense of transpersonal reverence, we find ourselves becoming useless in therapy. About all we can do is withdraw in wonder and awe at what this human being has become. But "awe" takes us right back to where we began!

REFERENCES

Bohart, A. C., O'Hara, M. M., & Leitner, L. M. (1998). Empirically violated treatments: Disenfranchisement of humanistic and other psychotherapies. *Psychotherapy Research, 8,* 141-157.

Buber, M. (1970). *I and thou.* New York: Charles Scribner.

Caplan, P. J. (1995). *They say you're crazy: How the world's most powerful psychiatrists decide who's normal.* Reading, MA: Addison-Wesley.

Chessick, R. (1974). *The technique and practice of intensive psychotherapy.* New York: Jason Aronson.

Epting, F. R. & Viney, L. L. (1999, July). Supervision in personal construct psychotherapy. Presented at the International Congress on Personal Construct Psychology, Berlin, Germany.

Farber, S. (1993). *Madness, heresy and the rumor of angels: The revolt against the mental health system.* Chicago: Open Court.

Faidley, A. J. (1993). ROLE relationships: A methodology for exploring shared universes of meaning. Unpublished doctoral dissertation, Miami University.

Faidley, A. J. & Leitner, L. M. (1993). *Assessing experience in psychotherapy: Personal construct alternatives.* Westport, CT: Praeger.

Faidley, A. J. & Leitner, L. M. (in press). The poetry of our lives: Symbolism in experiential personal construct psychotherapy. In J. Scheer (Ed.), *The person in society: Challenges to a constructivist theory.* Giessen, Germany: Psychosozial Verlag.

Honos-Webb, L. & Leitner, L. M. (in press). How DSM diagnoses damage: A client speaks. *Journal of Humanistic Psychology.*

Kelly, G. A. (1991a). *The psychology of personal constructs* (Vol. 1). London: Routledge. (Original published 1955)

Kelly, G. A. (1991b). *The psychology of personal constructs* (Vol. 2). London: Routledge. (Original published 1955)

Kutchins, H. & Kirk, S. A. (1997). *Making us crazy: DSM: The psychiatric Bible and the creation of mental disorders.* New York: The Free Press.

Laing, R. D. (1969). *The divided self.* New York: Penguin.

Landfield, A. W. (1976). A personal construct approach to suicidal behavior. In P. Slater (Ed.), *Explorations of intrapersonal space* (Vol. 1) (pp. 93-107). London: John Wiley.

Leitner, L. M. (1985). The terrors of cognition: On the experiential validity of personal construct theory. In D. Bannister (Ed.), *Issues and approaches in personal construct theory* (pp. 83-103). London: Academic.

Leitner, L. M. (1988). Terror, risk, and reverence: Experiential personal construct psychotherapy. *International Journal of Personal Construct Psychology, 1,* 261-272.

Leitner, L. M. (1995a). Dispositional assessment techniques in experiential personal construct psychotherapy. *Journal of Constructivist Psychology, 8,* 53-74.

Leitner, L. M. (1995b). Optimal therapeutic distance: A therapist's experience of personal construct psychotherapy. In R. Neimeyer & M. Mahoney (Eds.), *Constructivism in psychotherapy.* Washington, D.C.: American Psychological Association.

Leitner, L. M. (1997, July). Transference and countertransference in experiential personal construct psychotherapy. Presented at the International Congress on Personal Construct Psychology, Seattle, WA.

Leitner, L. M. (1999). Levels of awareness in experiential personal construct psychotherapy. *Journal of Constructivist Psychology, 12,* 239-252.

Leitner, L. M. (1999). Terror, numbness, panic, and awe: Experiential personal constructivism and panic. *The Psychotherapy Patient, 11*(1/2), 157-170.

Leitner, L. M. & Celentana, M. A. (1997). Constructivist therapy with serious disturbances. *The Humanistic Psychologist, 25,* 309-317.

Leitner, L. M. & Dill-Standiford, T. J. (1993). Resistance in experiential personal construct psychotherapy: Theoretical and technical struggles. In L. M. Leitner & N. G. M. Dunnett (Eds.), *Critical issues in personal construct psychotherapy* (pp. 135-155). Malabar, FL: Krieger.

Leitner, L. M. & Faidley, A. J. (1995). The awful, aweful nature of ROLE relationships. In G. Neimeyer & R. Neimeyer (Eds.), *Advances in personal construct psychology* (Vol. III) (pp. 291-314). Greenwich, CT: Praeger.

Leitner, L. M. & Faidley, A. J. (1999). Creativity in experiential personal construct psychotherapy. *Journal of Constructivist Psychology, 12,* 273-286.

Leitner, L. M., Faidley, A. J., & Celentana, M. A. (2000). Diagnosing human meaning making: An experiential constructivist approach. In R. Neimeyer & J. Raskin (Eds.), *Construction of Disorders: Meaning making frameworks for psychotherapy* (pp. 175-203). Washington, D.C.: American Psychological Association.

Leitner, L. M. & Guthrie, A. F. (1993). Validation of therapist interventions in psychotherapy: Clarity, ambiguity, subjectivity. *International Journal of Personal Construct Psychology, 6,* 281-294.

Leitner, L. M. & Pfenninger, D. T. (1994). Sociality and optimal functioning. *Journal of Constructivist Psychology 7,* 119-135.

Miller, I. (1996). Ethical and liability issues concerning invisible rationing. *Professional Psychology: Research and Practice, 27,* 583-587.

Rychlak, J. F. (1994). *Logical learning theory: A human teleology and its empirical support.* Lincoln: University of Nebraska Press.

Reflections on Mystery and Awe

David N. Elkins

SUMMARY. In this "Discussant's Response" to the foregoing papers, the author shares his own reactions and then underscores the importance of awe by quoting poets, mystics, writers, and scholars who understood that mystery is central to human life. *[Article copies available for a fee from The Haworth Document Delivery Service: 1-800-342-9678. E-mail address: <getinfo@haworthpressinc.com> Website: <http://www.HaworthPress. com> © 2001 by The Haworth Press, Inc. All rights reserved.]*

KEYWORDS. Therapeutic awe, HMOs, decisions, Lorca, mystics, religion, Buber, Maslow, Whitman, James, Rogers, Tillich, Frankl

Normally, the task of the discussant in a symposium is to critique the presentations in that critical, analytical way in which we have all been trained. But our goal here is different. In his proposal for this symposium, Kirk Schneider, our chairperson, said,

> Our aim in this symposium is to illuminate understanding of therapeutic awe, but also to have something of a freewheeling dialogue. As much

---

David N. Elkins, PhD, is a licensed clinical psychologist and tenured Professor of psychology in the Graduate School of Education and Psychology at Pepperdine University. In 1998-1999 he was president of the Humanistic Psychology Division of the American Psychological Association. His major interests are spirituality and the arts, especially poetry. He is author of *Beyond Religion: A Personal Program for Building a Spiritual Life Outside the Walls of Traditional Religion* (Quest Books, 1998).

Address correspondence to: David N. Elkins, Pepperdine University, Graduate School of Education and Psychology, 2151 Michelson Drive, Irvine, CA 92612.

[Haworth co-indexing entry note]: "Reflections on Mystery and Awe." Elkins, David N. Co-published simultaneously in *The Psychotherapy Patient* (The Haworth Press, Inc.) Vol. 11, No. 3/4, 2001, pp. 163-168; and: *Frightful Stages: From the Primitive to the Therapeutic* (ed: Robert B. Marchesani, and E. Mark Stern) The Haworth Press, Inc., 2001, pp. 163-168. Single or multiple copies of this article are available for a fee from The Haworth Document Delivery Service [1-800-342-9678, 9:00 a.m. - 5:00 p.m. (EST). E-mail address: getinfo@haworthpressinc.com].

as possible, we would like to "stretch the limits," both in terms of the contents of our talks, as well as in the dialogue that ensues following our talks. We would like to engage the audience in this exploratory dialogue as well, encouraging the most "far out," speculative, and intuitive reflections on the topic.

I suspect the most stifling thing I could do to kill a creative, "freewheeling dialogue" about awe would be to launch into an intellectual critique of these presentations. Conversely, perhaps the most helpful, enlivening thing I could do would be to share the thoughts, feelings, and images that have been stirred in me as I have thought about this symposium and listened to these presentations. So that's what I will do.

INITIAL REACTIONS TO A SYMPOSIUM ON AWE

My first reaction, when Kirk invited me to participate in this symposium, was something like this: "I agree that awe is an important topic, but can we really talk about it for two hours in a symposium at APA?" I wondered if we would be able to say anything stimulating about the topic. I wondered if anyone would show up to hear the presentation. As I look back on that reaction, I think I was reacting to the risk of talking about such a topic at APA. Awe is seldom talked about in psychology circles. It is almost never talked about at APA conventions!

Another early reaction I had could be worded as follows: "What a different model of psychotherapy is assumed by this symposium!" I thought of the therapeutic world we live in today in which managed care and HMOs are the dominant force. APA itself is developing guidelines consisting of standardized procedures for therapeutic intervention. Short-term, medical and mechanistic techniques are highly prized in our profession. I smiled to myself as I imagined writing a client progress report for a managed care company: "Client making excellent progress. Had two intense experiences of awe this past week. Anticipate more in near future."

BUILDING CATHEDRALS TO THE GLORY OF GOD

Then I began to think more seriously about this experience of awe. I remembered an old story about two brick layers who were helping build a church. A visitor asked one worker what he was doing and he grumpily replied, "I'm laying bricks. What does it look like I'm doing!" The visitor walked around to another part of the building and asked the second worker the same question. This worker stood, looked toward the heavens, and said, "I'm building a cathedral to the glory of God."

I wondered: do some therapists just lay bricks and do some build cathedrals to the glory of God? Do we forget in our therapeutic work that we are dealing with lives, with the very existences of human beings? Do we forget that clients will make decisions in our offices that will forever change their lives, that as a result of those decisions their lives will veer in completely new and unanticipated directions? Then I thought, "We *are* building cathedrals to God's glory. What an awesome privilege! What an awesome responsibility!"

THE SENSE OF MYSTERY AND AWE

Then I began to think about how important the sense of mystery and awe was to many of the scholars and writers I admire most. Quotations came flooding back into memory.

For example, I thought of the great Spanish poet and playwright Federico Garcia Lorca, who wrote at the bottom of one of his drawings, "Only mystery enables us to live, only mystery" (see Hirsch, 1999).

I thought of the German theologian Rudolph Otto (1961) and his book *The Idea of the Holy*. Otto did a phenomenological analysis of our encounters with the sacred, showing that awe is always a central component of such encounters. Otto also talked about the "energy of the numen" and how it ignited the souls of the mystics. He said this numinous experience is the core of all religion.

I thought of Mircea Eliade (1961) who was chair of the History of Religions Department at the University of Chicago for seventeen years and who wrote *The Sacred and the Profane*. Eliade spoke of these same awe-filled, mystical moments in life that Otto had described. Eliade called them "hierophanies," which literally means "something sacred shows itself to us." He believed these moments were qualitatively different from our everyday secular life, that in hierophanies we touch the truth, the really real.

I thought of that crazy poet and genius William Blake (1977), who said, "If the doors of perception were cleansed, we would see everything as it is, infinite" (p. 188).

I thought of Rumi, the great Sufi mystic of the thirteenth century, who would sometimes stay up all night with his community of dervishes, dancing, drinking wine, and reading poetry, hoping the Presence would appear. Rumi and Sufi mystics sought the experience of awe directly.

I thought of Martin Buber (1970) and his book *I and Thou*. Buber talked about the awe-filled experience of the I-Thou encounter. Not only do we have such experiences with other people, we also have these experiences in nature. As Buber said, we see a tree. We may notice its branches and leaves, even its beauty. But then sometimes, if we are fortunate, this I-It relationship falls away and we are drawn into a relational unity with the tree. This not only happens with trees, of course, but also with sunsets, oceans, mountains, and other things in nature. These events are always filled with awe.

I thought of Abraham Maslow (1968, 1976) and how he was almost obsessed with the realm of being and with those mystical, awe-filled moments in life that he called "peak experiences." Maslow wanted us to open our hearts to these experiences. He wanted education to include what he called "being cognition," viewing things under the aspect of eternity. In his longing to introduce students to this kind of knowing, Maslow once pointed out that you can teach a student to hear the sounds of a Beethoven quartet, but how do you teach the student to hear the *beauty* of those sounds?

I thought of Walt Whitman (1988), that poet so filled with the sense of mystery and awe. One of his poems seems to say it all.

> When I heard the learn'd astronomer,
> When the proofs, the figures, were ranged in columns before me,
> When I was shown the charts and diagrams, to add, divide, and measure them,
> When I sitting heard the astronomer where he lectured with much applause in the lecture-room,
> How soon unaccountable I became tired and sick,
> Till rising and gliding out I wander'd off by myself,
> In the mystical moist night-air, and from time to time,
> Look'd up in perfect silence at the stars. (p. 30)

I thought of William James (1982), who filled his book *The Varieties of Religious Experience* with stories of awe-filled encounters with the mystical and the sacred.

I thought of Carl Rogers (1989) who in his famous dialogue with theologian Paul Tillich said,

> I feel at times when I'm really being helpful to a client of mine, in those sort of rare moments where there is something approximating an I-Thou relationship between us, and when I feel that something significant is happening, then I feel as though I am somehow in tune with the forces in the universe or that forces are operating through me in regard to this helping relationship. . . . (p. 74)

And finally, I thought of one of the most touching stories of awe that I know. Viktor Frankl was my graduate professor. Frankl was imprisoned in the concentration camps of Hitler during World War II. His whole family was killed, including his 24-year-old wife. When Frankl was liberated in 1945 by the Allied Forces, he had no place to go. His family had been killed, the city where he had formerly lived was in ruins, Europe itself was decimated by the war. Frankl's heart was filled with despair. Then, in a deeply moving passage, Frank (1963) tells of a transforming experience of awe.

> One day, a few days after the liberation, I walked through the country past flowering meadows, for miles and miles, toward the market town near the camp. Larks rose to the sky and I could hear their joyous song. There was no one to be seen for miles around; there was nothing but the wide earth and sky and the larks' jubilation and the freedom of space. I stopped, looked around, and up to the sky–and then I went down on my knees. At that moment there was very little I knew of myself or of the world–I had but one sentence in mind–always the same: "I called to the Lord from my narrow prison and He answered me in the freedom of space."
>
> How long I knelt there and repeated this sentence memory can no longer recall. But I know that on that day, in that hour, my new life started. Step for step I progress, until again I became a human being. (pp. 141-42)

CONCLUSION

So I have come to know, once again, that awe is indeed important, not only in psychotherapy but in all of life. Awe is a lightning bolt that marks in memory those moments when the doors of perception are cleansed and we see with startling clarity what is truly important in life. Moments of awe may be the most important, transformative experiences of life.

Perhaps Federico Garcia Lorca was right: "Only mystery enables us to live, only mystery."

REFERENCES

Otto, R. (1961). *The idea of the holy.* New York: Oxford University Press.

Eliade, M. (1961). *The sacred and the profane.* New York: Harper & Row.

Blake, W. (1977). The marriage of heaven and hell. In A. Ostriker (Ed.), *William Blake: The complete poems* (p. 188). New York: Penguin Books.

Buber, M. (1970). *I and thou.* New York: Charles Scribner's Sons.

Maslow, A. (1976). *Religions, values, and peak experiences.* New York: Penguin Books.

Maslow, A. (1968). *Toward a psychology of being.* New York: Van Nostrand Reinhold.

Whitman, W. (1988). When I heard the learn'd astronomer. In L.B. Hopkins (Ed.), *Voyages: Poems by Walt Whitman* (p. 30). New York: Harcourt Brace Jovanovich.

James, W. (1982). *The varieties of religious experience.* New York: Penguin Books.

Rogers, C. (1989). Paul Tillich. In H. Kirschenbaum & V. L. Henderson (Eds.), *Carl Rogers: Dialogues.* (p. 31). Boston: Houghton Mifflin.

Frankl, V. (1963). *Man's search for meaning.* New York: Pocket Books.

Hirsch, E. (1999). The duende. *The American Poetry Review,* 28(4)13-21.

On Anguish and Other Frightful Moments in the Process of Self-Discovery

Scott Churchill

SUMMARY. Presented in the form of a journal, this article takes a heuristic approach to existential "fear and trembling" by focusing on the concerns and associations that awakened the author one night on the dawn of a new year. Presented in a raw, stream-of-consciousness style (complete with defensive intellectualizations), the narrative circles around issues of anguish, panic, and personal responsibility, all in relation to interpersonal life. At once a confession and a personal exploration, it is, in retrospect, a seeking that has not yet found its destination–it is perhaps something akin to what the Germans call *"unterwegs"* *("on the way")* toward an understanding of self and other. *[Article copies available for a fee from The Haworth Document Delivery Service: 1-800-342-9678. E-mail address: <getinfo@haworthpressinc.com> Website: <http://www.HaworthPress.com>   © 2001 by The Haworth Press, Inc. All rights reserved.]*

KEYWORDS. Unrest, regret, panic, anxiety, symptoms, remorse, culpability, abandonment, insomnia, paralysis

---

Scott Churchill earned his doctorate in clinical phenomenological psychology at Duquesne University. He is currently Chairman and Associate Professor of Psychology at the University of Dallas, where he has been teaching for 20 years. An active member of the executive board of the APA's Division 32 (Humanistic Psychology), his professional focus is on the development of phenomenological and hermeneutic methodologies; his interests vary from clinical psychology to film studies to research on the social behavior of primates. He has taught graduate psychology courses at Duquesne University and Pacifica Graduate Institute and has been film critic for the Irving Community Television Network since 1984.

[Haworth co-indexing entry note]: "On Anguish and Other Frightful Moments in the Process of Self-Discovery." Churchill, Scott. Co-published simultaneously in *The Psychotherapy Patient* (The Haworth Press, Inc.) Vol. 11, No. 3/4, 2001, pp. 169-180; and: *Frightful Stages: From the Primitive to the Therapeutic* (ed: Robert B. Marchesani, and E. Mark Stern) The Haworth Press, Inc., 2001, pp. 169-180. Single or multiple copies of this article are available for a fee from The Haworth Document Delivery Service [1-800-342-9678, 9:00 a.m. - 5:00 p.m. (EST). E-mail address: getinfo@haworthpressinc.com].

I establish myself as a person in so far as I assume responsibility for my acts and so behave as a real being.

–Gabriel Marcel

You feel you are hedged in; you dream of escape; but beware of mirages. Do not run or fly away in order to get free: rather dig in the narrow place which has been given you; you will find God there and everything. . . . If you fly away from yourself, your prison will run with you and will close in because of the wind of your flight; if you go deep down into yourself it will disappear in paradise.

–Gustave Thibon

Ferrara, Italy: January 2, 2000

Waking up suddenly in the middle of the night, in the dark, in one of those moments when you are alone with yourself–especially in a foreign land, jet-lagged, and on the dawn of a new millennium–this qualifies as one of those moments of "uncanniness" where you can find yourself face to face with your predicament in life. It is in these pristine hours of a day which has not yet begun that one can experience a profound sense of anguish in the face of those circumstances or "facticities" which, for the moment, are held at a distance even as they continue to beleaguer one's soul. In the silence of a still morning, there is a momentary suspension of one's daily projects and pressures, occasioning a stream of consciousness in which one takes stock of oneself. Such reflection might be peaceful, it might be angst-ridden, or it might even culminate in a disturbance of oneself to the point where an unwelcome restlessness expresses itself in the form of cardiac arrhythmia (or at the very least occasions one's getting out of bed, as if in an effort to re-establish one's bond with the world by engaging in some simple task such as getting a glass of water).

What is it that one faces in such moments of nocturnal uneasiness? (I am choosing here to reflect on my own nighttime occurrences of anguish, to provide some concrete reference point for my reflections, as these are more familiar to me–but it could easily as well be a lapse into a fearful reverie in the middle of the day that would provoke a similar foray into the deepest concerns and worries that trouble one's soul.) Thanks to depth psychology, I am able to be present to both the current distress and its deeper significance contemporaneously, insofar as I understand that whatever it is that troubles me so profoundly that I cannot go back to sleep must be a symptom of a more pervasive concern, an ontological unrest, that defines me even as I lose myself in waking life in my mundane world of concern.

Tonight, the occasion for my being unsettled is that I am experiencing the weight of earlier choices that now have become a part of my destiny, so to speak; facticity has its ugly way of bearing down upon oneself, even when one is an existentialist at heart! It would be easier if I could simply experience regret; but it is too late for regret–or perhaps too soon. (That is, regret would seem to require conscious action in the first place, and what I am entering into here are those actions which lie on the frontier between choice that knows itself as choice, and a species of choice that Sartre aptly termed "bad faith.") Without the determination to follow through on one's resolutions to change, one can only stand in anguish in the face of the course of events that one has set into motion, and which one is perhaps too weak to alter. "The way out is through the door–why is it that no one will use the door?" I suppose the answer to that question is in knowing that we have made our bed, and now we must sleep in it. This is not the first time in my life that I have found myself unable to live from day to day without a lurking and disarmingly dreadful sense of apprehension. I can recall more carefree times, when all I needed to think about was how to dress for class that day, what inspiring ideas I might share with my students, which movie to go to tonight, and what book to read out by the pool. But at some point in life other responsibilities enter the picture, responsibilities that are our choices, even when they are not our obligations.

As I enter this new millennium (it is 5 a.m. on the 2nd of January as I write this from my bedside in Italy) with a sense of resolve to right those things that have been wrong in my life and pray to discover a renewed sense of happiness, I am unable to fall back to sleep, because my soul is burdened by a situation that I left 6,000 miles away, but which nonetheless is closer to me now than the pillow is to my face. Indeed, the possibility of happiness right here and now, during these next 10 days, is tainted by the weight of both my immediate past and by the ever-widening horizons of past experiences that fall into relief as each life context invoked in this morning's early reverie becomes figural against yet another, earlier-established ground of experience. In the end, the free association here becomes a chain of signifiers each invoking another set of circumstances all seeming to bear the same structure.

So as to free myself here from the specific concerns that make up my current dis-ease, in order to see through to the more invariant nature of my own peculiar set of personal storylines, I will look to what has been signified in the occasionally disturbing nocturnal awakenings stretching over a decade now, to try to find some common center to them. In all of them I find most distinctively a sense of anguish which, even before it ever escalates to the point of a full blown panic attack, nonetheless exists in nascent form as a profound sense of disturbance in my more immediate interpersonal sphere.

By this I mean that it doesn't have much to do with practical concerns and worries, such as any impending or already sustained failures in investment activities, for example–although the very word "investment" strikes me as appropriate here in a more existential sense, insofar as it seems to be only those interpersonal situations in which I find myself heavily invested, that have the potential to provoke such dread-ridden streams of consciousness as I am experiencing this morning.

Likewise, my anxieties at midlife concerning career decisions are not of the kind that are capable of provoking panic (thank goodness!). No, the terror of which I speak is something that swells up out of the depths of one's more intimate personal life, for no matter how much one might console oneself or divert oneself in daily life from *angst* (e.g., by calling to mind all of one's predominantly happy adjustments and accomplishments in the interpersonal field), there lurks heavily upon one's soul in such moments of troubled sleep, one or more particular faces–indeed, the faces of those persons either already or potentially intertwined in one's particular destiny.

I see two primary vicissitudes of such anguished moments as I am experiencing now. Associated with the first is the nurturing image of my mother (for whom I thank God that she is still here with me, to continue guiding me), and how she would be affected by the consequences of my more troublesome behaviors–i.e., she is the one who taught me right from wrong, to live in moderation, to "eat three good meals a day, get a full night's sleep, and never put off until tomorrow what you can accomplish today; stay away from drugs and other dangerous activity, and be thankful that you have your health." So when several years ago I went through a period of panic attacks, what they signified to me was in part my sole responsibility for having put myself in the position that resulted in my cardiac arrhythmia. All of the medical "explanations" and reassurances were no relief from further anxiety, for like a Sartrean anti-hero, I was acutely aware that it was not my heart's beta contractions, but rather a long series of situational choices (and ironically self-destructive behaviors) that had led to the point where I found myself. I could find no solace in the sudden and peculiar "fact" that one out of ten people was allegedly being diagnosed with panic disorders–this was too obviously a false way of pretending that somehow all these panic-stricken individuals were victims of some "syndrome," as if the sheer pervasiveness of the malady were evidence of its origins outside the human realm of freedom and choice.

So the first form of anguish comes to me in the face of the reassuring but at the same time "concerned" image of my mother (and implicitly my father who passed away almost 10 years ago)–for it was they who gave me, not only life, but the rules by which to live it. And if I had been able to act throughout my adult life as though they were still there with me, guiding me along, then for sure I would not have put myself in those situations that could occasion terrifying panic (and which at one time even led to my carrying around a heart monitor for a month). These frightful moments made me aware that I was to blame-that I had been choosing all along the course of my own destiny (which might even include an early death). And in my worrisome sleeplessness and attacks of arrhythmia, I conjured up saddened images of my mother and father (as well as my sister and brother), in the face of whom I was obviously feeling ashamed for all the lapses of good judgment (drinking, smoking, stress, staying up too late) that had created or at least contributed to my current "medical condition."

It was this experience that more than anything else brought home the insight that a medical condition must also be treated as a symptom, and not just an explanation; a dis-ease of the soul, and not just a factual state of affairs of the objective body. Today we are prone to confuse description with explanation: each newly identified psychological syndrome, rather than simply describing manifest conditions, also becomes in a curious and circular way its own explanation: the *reason* I can't concentrate is *because* I "have" ADHD (rather than the diagnosis simply describing the *fact* that I do not concentrate). So, when someone like myself goes to his doctor with symptoms of panic, they are *explained* as the occurrence of panic disorder. But this is wrong. These symptoms point to something else that we prefer not to look at, something else that does not show itself to the physician–namely, our own sense of culpability.

The second vicissitude alluded to earlier is in fact what often serves as a prelude to the first, which I shall now refer to as *an anguished remorse in the face of who I might have been (or might have become)*. That is, what I have described up to now is an anguish about the possibilities that have been lost on account of who I have chosen to be, what I have chosen to do with myself, and with whom I have chosen to involve myself. This can even be the "shadow side" of our greatest achievements: my life in academia has been infused with all the energies that might otherwise have gone into building a home life with someone I love–and had I earlier set up my priorities differently, the anxieties that I now feel in the face of my (loss of) possibilities might not be what they are. (Of course, I would have then a different set of anxieties to write about!) But, more than simply "in principle" alluding to those possibilities negated necessarily by life's choices, I am referring here to those possibilities that we might have nonetheless actualized, were it not for our less admirable choices. My choice to incarnate myself as an enthusiastic and accessible college professor is not what has occasioned my lack of good habits. I may have forsaken other life projects (marriage, family life) for the sake of my own style of *being* an academic; but my career is indeed something that I am proud of–and of which my parents were always proud, too. So the real culprit exposed here is not one's career choice but lifestyle choices that affect our potential for further growth.

I am still circling around the particular issue that is disquieting to me at this very moment, and that is the issue pertaining to a second kind of dread: *a dread in the face of pain I may have caused in another's life.* When I first awoke this morning to the sound of peaceful snoring from the other room, I became consumed by my recollection of last night's phone call to someone very dear to me, who had been deeply hurt by my not stopping to think that this trip during winter recess which I had already planned over a year ago (indeed, I have been dreaming about taking such a trip overseas for several years now), how this trip would nonetheless leave this person feeling alone and abandoned, and not having been taken into account.

The anxieties described earlier all pertained to what I have done to myself; this second variation pertains to how I have affected others. How do I live with myself when someone is telling me that I am causing them pain because I don't care *enough* about them, or won't make them the center of my life? It doesn't matter that in such circumstances the other person might already have been in significant emotional pain long before you met. For once you have entered into a relationship with someone, this relationship then becomes the inevitable (and often unwitting) context for subsequent pain and disharmony. You cannot escape from the fact that even in your attempts to rescue others from their own particular sense of unhappiness or abandonment, you are setting yourself up to be the next one to hurt them. Indeed, long before such a relationship might ever end (and, at this point, I must say that I am doubtful that such relationships ever truly "end"), abandonment will have become a long-established and much troubled theme in the relationship, perhaps even the defining subtext of each newly occurring strain within the relationship: the other now feels abandoned by you, ironically, the very person who at the outset provided a haven of comfort for the other. This irony becomes the context for what I will refer to as *an anguished remorse in the face of what I cannot do over again, cannot take back.* Once this anguish settles into one's spirit, all of one's simple plans become complicated by what one now experiences as everything from guilt-ridden oversights to unwelcome obligations. (In such situations, it seems that what you once gave freely to the other is now not only expected, but anticipated with a sense of entitlement.) A heart-wrenching anguish finally emerges when it appears that there is no exit. Unable to "use the door," what is left is only a kind of resignation that eats away at one's own existence.

*   *   *

January 3, 2000

So far I have neatly evaded a direct reflection upon my troubled sleep last night. On the one hand, in tackling this article that I had promised to write, I did not want to lapse merely into self-referential detail (for reasons of both privacy and confidentiality, I have remained hovering at a safe distance from the actual storyline itself). On the other hand, I realize that what I have written so far is nonetheless a very personal statement, no matter how abstractly I have rendered it. Perhaps this morning, a day later, and after having been up all night, I can try to bring some closure to the can of worms opened when I began this essay a day ago.

Alas, my first move is again an avoidant one: a stream of consciousness adumbrating different sets of circumstances, each with its own moments of dread, in order to attempt to see through to their common structure as well as their differences. I realize upon reflection that only a certain degree of my own anxieties pertains, on the one hand, to a sense of *guilt* or responsibility for what I have done that might have affected someone else rather badly. *Panic* sets in, on the other hand, at the thought of being exposed, as well as when one has an immediate sense that one might be "done in" or "done for." The difference, in fact, between panic and anguish would seem to be whether or not the situation seems to oneself to be a matter of survival. One panics when one really believes that one is about to die (or even just lose one's position in life). One anguishes over those choices that one must necessarily carry to one's death. (Perhaps this is why Kierkegaard wrote of the "sickness unto death.")

What defines "life or death" varies idiosyncratically from individual to individual. Let me give an example of how something that begins with good intent can lead to a kind of disastrous and pervasive sense of doom. Some years ago I was subpoenaed to give a deposition as a kind of "character witness" for a friend going through a divorce. I soon realized to my chagrin, however, that the questions I would be asked were more aimed at the defamation of the plaintiff in the case, my friend's new wife. I was being warned by other close friends that I would be subject to all kinds of cross-examination that would be aimed to destroy my credibility as a person, and that would lead into areas of my life that best remained private. I soon developed acute anxiety, escalating into full-blown panic attacks (although I have never liked this term to describe what I experienced–it was more like an intense *fright*). In retrospect, my concerns regarding the deposition were only a precipitating factor here; there is also the issue of my whole lifestyle at this moment in time–bad sleeping habits, overindulgences, constant worries, all leading up to what could otherwise seem like an entirely isolated symptom: a mysterious disturbance in my pulse. This first took the form of a slightly elevated heartbeat, one that could create a sense of flushing, and even a feeling of not being a part of the situation I was in (e.g., sitting in a movie theater, or at a meeting, I would find myself unable to concentrate–as though everything were taking place "out there" while I was secretly suffering something but unaware of what it might really be). Eventually I would find myself noticing what I would later learn was called "palpitations"–a benign-sounding term for a most frightening experience!

Arrhythmias were causing me to take my pulse constantly; I could not sleep at night, and when I did, I experienced terrifying dreams of sinking into some kind of sludge, and dying by grotesque heart attacks. I felt all alone, in need of a guiding hand. It was at this moment that a dear friend and trusted colleague stepped in, recognizing intuitively that I was in need of some help. What I later received when I returned to Dallas and sought medical consultation was three months of Xanax therapy (for which, at the time, I was grateful)–followed by rebound insomnia (but fortunately no rebound depression).

I had been shaken to the core by my fears–initially it was my imagination of what it would be like to be alone under attack in a legal cross-examination (my worries here spread also to concern about others who might be implicated or otherwise hurt). Beyond this, there was a concern for where I had placed myself in life–and those moments alone with myself when I felt "unsure" to the point of being lost. The arrhythmia was itself this *being-shaken*. It was a profound confusion, not knowing what to do, which way to turn, until this indecisiveness and uncontrollable thought patterns filtered down to the level of the body, to the very heart of my being, which itself was racing and out of control, hesitating, speeding up–an urgent sign of calamity. The tail was now wagging the dog, as I could not control my panic, I could only suffer it.[1]

It was indeed a feeling that extended far beyond the circumstance of the legal deposition itself, to the wider context of a particular social subworld of which I had become involved (initially at a distance), and also the more immediate context of a painfully dysfunctional relationship I was suffering, being caught up in someone else's "borderline syndrome" (I recognize the need here to re-assign the quotation marks: I should rather say that I was living within the context of "someone else's" borderline syndrome. Putting it this way is a way of acknowledging how at the time I experienced it as *the other's* dysfunctional history, while admitting to myself now that it had become *my* dysfunction as well, wherever it might have originated.) I had been absorbing on an almost daily basis the outwardly projected verbal abuses my friend had once suffered from her own mother. I was trying to help her, but the "cure" worked both ways–like a "Kentucky (cured) ham," I was absorbing the very emotional dynamics that I was otherwise trying to help free her from. There were moments when I even considered the possibility of leaving my own apartment, my job, my city, all to get free of this situation. There was also a strong sense of culpability–others were telling me this was my "co-dependence" (I knew better than to fall into the nominal fallacy: naming it would not yield much insight into it). In any case, for reasons that amount to a separate story, which I will not elaborate, I chose to stay in my situation and attempt to weather the storm.

In the end, it changed me. I cannot say necessarily for the better. And though I continue to care about (and from time to time find myself continuing to *care for*) my friend, I have been generally avoidant of any kind of deep involvement ever since. Behaviorists teach that fear conditioning can occur with one trial. It has taken me some years to begin to feel free again.

*   *   *

So this time, I find myself in a situation where I have discovered that the person with whom I was finally learning to explore new ground indeed had her own set of vulnerabilities: not feeling loved at home when she was growing up, currently feeling abandoned by the few friends to whom she had really come to feel close. And then I entered the scene, someone who would listen to her and spend time with her, someone whom she could trust. It wasn't long before she would begin talking about her anticipations of the next year, the "precious little time" we would have together before her career plans would separate her from me. I was initially taken aback when after only several weeks of spending time together, there was already a projected plan for spending the whole next year together–indeed, after having just completed several months of back therapy and frightening medical diagnostic procedures (chasing shadows from a series of sonograms and CAT scans), I was now beginning to feel I could look ahead to some "open horizons"–and already my next year was being planned for me! I discovered once more that I did not have the strength to protest. (In any case, I had not ruled out such a possibility, and I did not want to create a disturbance in the relationship, so I just went along with it, even if I felt not completely at ease with the way in which my tacit compliance constituted a complicity in the projected future plans.) Soon, travel plans that I had long ago made and committed myself to were creating some discontentment. At this point in the relationship, I was spending a lot of time worrying about my friend's physical and emotional pains, which I learned she had been internalizing for years. I was the only person who knew the extent of her pain and unhappiness.

Eventually I found myself stymied as to how to help her get past or get over her sense of rejection at having been "left" by significant others in her past. Worse yet, I was beginning to notice ways in which disturbances in our current relationship began to bear the mark of "transferences" from her past. Just before leaving on my current trip overseas, I would learn that she felt hurt that I didn't "need" her the way she needed me, because, she said, if she weren't there, my whole world would not fall apart. Although later she would say I took this too literally, it did not take much to interpret this as a kind of "reversal"-for, indeed, whenever I was away, it seemed to her that her world *was* falling apart. Saying goodbye, even on the phone, became excruciating.

(I almost can't bear writing this, but I feel it is necessary in order to give at least some palpable sense to the weight that I am feeling right now as I lie here in bed. What I was referring to at the start of the essay as a heavy "facticity" is precisely this state of affairs, within the horizon of my previous mistakes.)

So how does one become free from such an entanglement? I value this person, would like to be her friend, would like to try to help make her life a little happier-but I cannot suffer the responsibility of being her only lifeline. My heart just skipped a beat (for the first time in months) as I write this. It is my fault for letting it go on, but it is too late to cry over spilt milk, and she may be on the verge of an emotional collapse that was imminent long before I met her-only now, it would be perceived as "on my account." So I feel paralyzed.

Yes, a paralysis-an existential paralysis. This is what beleaguers me. Perhaps my death dreams five years ago were an expression of this kind of paralysis-not being able to move, dreaming that I was sinking into some thick sludge, unable to cry out for help-only a howling moan being emitted from my mouth as my heart, beating alarmingly hard in my chest, caused my rib cage to break open like a bird's nest pushed inside-out from behind.

*   *   *

I lay awake in these wee hours while others are asleep, their bodies and souls at rest. I lay here, staring into dark space, alone with my anxieties, running my tongue behind my teeth, feeling the crowns, wondering like a Woody Allen character about the possibly decaying tissue inside one of the capped teeth that has been acting up, wondering how long before I break another tooth or have to start in with root canals. (Yes, indeed, along with paralysis of the soul comes the symbolism of castration and Thanatos!) My belly seems hopelessly like my dad's now, and the age spots beginning to appear on my hands and face, the hint of vericose veins just under the skin, the slight thinning of my ever-graying hair, the stiffness of my joints, and even what might seem to be an untimely waning of my sexual appetite, all signal to me a rather sudden demise of the Peter Pan persona I had rather successfully managed to sustain for the past quarter century.

Kierkegaard wrote in *The Sickness Unto Death* that the despair of necessity is due to the lack of possibility. (It was his converse form of despair-namely, the despair of possibility due to the lack of necessity-that had beleaguered me throughout my twenties and thirties. Each the "shadow-side" of the other, these two forms of despair, working together in the "alchemy" of my soul life, probably resulted in my never settling down.) But now these themes of anguish and despair all start coming together. At the same time, I am encouraged by Sartre's words that "the self which I am depends upon the self which I am not yet, to the exact extent that the self which I am not yet does *not* depend upon the self which I am."[2] (In other words, there is no determinism in human life, but only a "being-towards-possibilities.") This offers at least a point in the direction of a way out. But what has come together here is my realization that my fears are centered in the present as a present that could possibly rob me of my future–a present that bears the inescapable weight of my own past as well as the past of others who are dear to me–and a present that I am nonetheless fully responsible for getting myself into.

* * *

March 31, 3000

I have let my earlier reflections "sit" (while winter has turned into spring), and find myself anguishing now over its completion, or lack thereof. I am having trouble letting it go; indeed, gentle reminders from my Editor notwith-standing, I do not *want* to let it go–at least not in its present unfinished form. But, alas, I realize that like Kaspar Hauser's unfinished story (which he relates on his death bed, and which strangely enough seems to be complete in itself, even if he himself did not think so), my own confession comes full circle to where I stand now, and bears witness to my willingness to pursue these matters further.

"Thus," writes a wise mentor and friend, *"it seems to me that this experience is introductory . . . as if you have been put on notice (have put yourself on notice) that you are going to have to do something, about . . . You are looking for that part of the world that will make the anguish go away, if only you would attend to it. It is occurring to you, as you shop around through your life's situations, that THIS is the indecision that is most central. It is as if you are willing to die, except that you will have been a teacher, a son, a lover, a psychologist, but none of them sufficiently to justify personal peace, an answer to the anguish, and so you are even more willing to keep living, but who, which SCOTT, is to forge ahead? All of them have something; but doing them all is what you have done. Is it time, not to be more, but to be less–less strung out among these personae, each of which alone looks strangely like an indulgence.*

"I speak of this experience as 'introductory' seriously, for notions of a final significance to your life as a whole are certainly premature, but signifi-cance aside, that part of the world that deserves your attention, now, in the face of bodily, pedagogical, touristical, sexual, philosophical ongoingness, that choice about who to be now, after all the rest has proved to be not enough, continues to await you."

NOTES

1. One generally assumes that the heart runs on its own time–and perhaps this is what led physicians to "explain" my panic attacks as "simple" PACs (premature atrial contractions) which, if I continued to worry about them, might have led to the much more dangerous PVCs (premature ventricular contractions). But in fact I have learned that the heart does not run on "its own" time, but rather on *my* time. It is *I* who set the course of my daily rhythms, and hence my heart, like a dog's tail, follows the lead of its owner. And yet, once the pathological PACs begin, they do take on a life of their own, and one finds oneself suddenly intolerant of chocolate, caffeine, tea, etc. Cardiac arrhythmia attacks one as one awakens at some ungodly hour, feeling melancholic to begin with, and then out of nowhere comes this "... boom ... boom ... boom ... boom ... B-Boom ... boom ... boom ... boom ... boom ... B-boom ... B-boom ....BOOM BOOM ...... boom ... boom ..." and one has this sickening feeling that the heart is going to suddenly start fibrillating–or worse, stop altogether. One has at this point definitely "lost control" of one's own heart, and if in the ensuing panic one calls someone on the telephone just to hear the reassuring voice of a person one trusts, what one does NOT want to hear is a casual dismissal of the symptom–nor does one want to hear a sense of alarm, or disappointment, or a suggestion that maybe you had better drive yourself to the hospital (how can you even think of sitting up in bed, much less driving, with an arrhythmic heartbeat!). What one needs is a confident voice saying, "You are going to be all right, your heart will start beating regularly again in just a moment, everything is going to be fine, I am on my way over right now, I'll get you some water...." What, at least in my own case, was almost always the thing that would "save" me was the fact that someone cared enough to come right over and help, and sometimes the moment they left the arrhythmia would kick in again. So I learned right away that there was a curious interpersonal horizon involved in this experience.

2. *Being and Nothingness*, p. 69 (emphasis added). (New York: Washington Square Press, 1943/1956).

I'm Not Crazy,
They Are Coming Around with Guns!

Charles T. Tart

SUMMARY. This experience strikingly demonstrated to me how my mind (and minds in general) can distort information, especially when strong emotions are involved. Interviewing people about unusual experiences made me more sensitive to distinguishing what happened to people from their feelings about it.

KEYWORDS. Consciousness, meditation, violence, telepathy, Patty Hearst, panic, fright, shame, craziness, sensitivity

The late 1960s and early 1970s were exciting times for those of us interested in the nature of the human mind. Psychedelic drugs, eastern religions, new research on the nature of dreams, biofeedback, and other developments had given us new ways to look at and experiment with our own minds, but the

---

Charles T. Tart, PhD, is Core Faculty at the Institute of Transpersonal Psychology and Professor Emeritus of Psychology at UC Davis. He is internationally known for research with altered states, transpersonal psychology, and parapsychology. His 13 books include two classics, *Altered States of Consciousness* and *Transpersonal Psychologies*. Two recent books, *Waking Up* and *Living the Mindful Life*, synthesized Buddhist, Sufi, and Gurdjieffian mindfulness training ideas with modern psychology. His latest book, *Body Mind Spirit: Exploring the Parapsychology of Spirituality*, explores the scientific foundation of transpersonal psychology to show it is possible to be both a scientist and a spiritual seeker.

[Haworth co-indexing entry note]: "I'm Not Crazy, They Are Coming Around with Guns!" Tart, Charles T. Co-published simultaneously in *The Psychotherapy Patient* (The Haworth Press, Inc.) Vol. 11, No. 3/4, 2001, pp. 181-185; and: *Frightful Stages: From the Primitive to the Therapeutic* (ed: Robert B. Marchesani, and E. Mark Stern) The Haworth Press, Inc., 2001, pp. 181-185.

few of us working on scientific understandings of the mind largely worked in isolation. The too few meetings that brought us together were often the high points of the year.

In the spring of 1973, I attended one of the first Council Grove Conferences, dedicated to understanding the new developments in consciousness. Held at White Memorial Camp, an isolated church camp on the plains of Kansas, near the town of Council Grove, these unique conferences brought together people from all over the country who were interested in expanding human potentials, in understanding and developing some extraordinary things we could do with our minds if we could only transcend our ordinary limits. Council Grove is a good place for that kind of conference. There is something about the vastness of the plains and the wind sweeping in from vast distances that simultaneously humbles a person, yet says, "Think big!"

The Conference was a heady mixture of science and mysticism, with lectures by Indian yogis and American Indian medicine men following sober scientific reports on brain wave control and new techniques for self-healing. I had been studying various aspects of the human mind for many years, and came away inspired and stimulated with new ideas. Little did I realize that the Conference was to start a chain of events that would demonstrate one of the potentials of the mind to me and a friend in a frightening and vivid way, a way that was much more than just an idea.

A highlight of the Conference for me was meeting Terry Alexander (pseudonym), a bright young psychologist who was not only just getting his PhD in psychology from one of America's leading universities, but who had spent years personally studying meditation in India. Terry's combination of intellectual and experiential knowledge of an exciting subject like meditation was unique, and we had a lot to talk about. There is never enough time at conferences, though, so I asked him to let me know when he would be in Berkeley, California, where I lived, so we could continue our talks.

It was eight months before Terry got out to Berkeley, but he finally called me in February. We arranged for me to pick him up the next evening, February fourth, about nine o'clock. He was staying with friends in the same house that housed the Institute for the Study of Consciousness at 2924 Benvenue Avenue. The Institute, founded by Arthur Young, a well-known inventor, was a place I knew of as a developing center for scientists who had become interested in understanding consciousness, although I had not had a chance to visit it yet.

I knew the area, though, one of those lovely Berkeley residential neighborhoods of tree-lined streets, lovely old Victorians, and big brown-shingled houses that created the architectural style known as Berkeley brownshingle.

Terry mentioned that there would be a meeting going on in the front of the house when I arrived, and rather than disturb it, why didn't I come around to the kitchen door in the rear? We would then go out to a coffee shop and talk. That was fine, and I looked forward to our meeting.

The next evening I left my home in the northern part of Berkeley and drove south on San Pablo Avenue, a main thoroughfare, and planned to then turn east up Ashby Avenue, another main thoroughfare which intersected Benvenue. I was driving up San Pablo Avenue. As I approached my turn on to Ashby Avenue, I lost track of what I had been thinking about and instead found myself thinking about bad neighborhoods with criminal gangs in them. I thought that was silly: I was going to a nice section of Berkeley, not to some ghetto. The thought not only persisted, it quickly built into a frightening set of obsessions about being beaten up, about gangs of people with guns, shooting, violence, and the conviction that I would be mistaken for a burglar and shot when I walked between the houses to meet Terry at the kitchen door. I became very frightened and wanted to turn the car around and drive away as fast as possible. The closer I got to Benvenue Avenue, the worse I felt!

Simultaneously with my panic and obsession with being shot and beaten up, I felt intensely ashamed and embarrassed: I had to be crazy to feel like this! There was absolutely no reason for any normal person to feel this way! Had I only been fooling myself all these years, thinking I was normal, while underneath I was as crazy and sick as some of the psychotic patients I had studied? The psychologist part of my mind diagnosed me as having a paranoid schizophrenic attack of high intensity, and the outlook for my future wasn't very good if I was this crazy underneath! I was even more acutely embarrassed because I had spent years working on understanding my own mind through various kinds of psychotherapeutic, psychological, and spiritual growth techniques, yet it looked as if I was crazier than when I started!

The fear kept intensifying, but I fought it. I pulled over twice, preparatory to making a U-turn to drive back home, but each time I pulled back out and kept going. I absolutely refused to surrender to this craziness! Finally I reached Benvenue Avenue, turned onto it, saw roughly where 2924 was, and looked for a parking place. Parking was difficult. I drove several blocks down Benvenue looking, finally found a place, parked and walked a couple of blocks back to meet Terry. I was still quite frightened and I looked into every shadow and parked car, and between houses, looking for gangs or an ambush. I avoided the few people on the street as much as possible.

Much to my relief, Terry was waiting out in front of the house, so I didn't have to go though the alley between the houses! We said hello, chatted as we walked back to my car, and drove off to a coffee shop that was a couple of miles away. I actively stopped myself from thinking about my experience, for while the fear had subsided, I still felt ashamed of myself. Talking to Terry distracted me from my obsession with gangs and guns and violence, so my fear finally faded away completely. Naturally I didn't say anything to Terry about it: he was still a new friend and a respected colleague, and I would have hesitated to tell even my best friend about this crazy, shameful side of my mind.

Terry went back to the East Coast, and I thought no more about (repressed?) my "crazy spell" until a letter from him a week later brought it all back. After mentioning a few things of professional interest, he told me of a personal experience that he hadn't told to me the night we met because it seemed shameful to him. While he was waiting for me in front of the Institute, he started feeling paranoid, worrying about people with guns and getting shot! He too felt pretty silly and ashamed. He was relieved when I arrived and we left for the coffee shop.

So, the plot thickened. Had I been tuning in to Terry's mental state through some kind of telepathy? Was he tuning in to mine?

The next sentence in his letter was the real shock, though. Had I known that the heiress Patty Hearst had been kidnapped, just down the street, a few minutes after we had left?

I had not had a brief excursion into insanity, nor had Terry. Some kind of ESP was being used by the unconscious parts of our minds, and it was trying to warn us of real danger!

As I fought off panic and Terry felt paranoid a few minutes before nine, three members of the Symbionese Liberation Army, the SLA, had already kidnapped Peter Benenson, a mathematician at Berkeley's famous Lawrence Radiation Laboratory. He had gone grocery shopping at the Berkeley Co-operative Shopping Center on Shattuck Avenue, in the north end of town where I was coming from. A later newspaper interview with former SLA member Bill Harris (Oakland Tribune, Oct. 16, 1988) revealed that the SLA members had been standing in the Co-op grocery store parking lot for some time planning to steal a car, looking over cars as they drove by.

Benenson was the opportune victim. As he was unloading groceries from his car in his driveway, he was seized from behind by two men and a woman who had followed him. They threw him onto the back floor of his car and threatened that if he didn't stay down, they would kill him. The two men each carried an automatic rifle containing cyanide-tipped bullets, the woman waved a .38 automatic pistol. Benenson was in a state of terror for some time, as his car was driven around while he crouched on the floor. There was indeed plenty of fear and a gang with guns around for me and Terry to pick up on!

I drove up and down Benvenue Avenue after the SLA had kidnapped Peter Benenson, looking for a parking place. Benvenue is a street where it is always difficult to find a parking place, but, as I learned from later newspaper accounts, one or two other cars filled with armed SLA members were parked on Benvenue close to 2603 when Patty was kidnapped at 9:20 p.m. Were they already there as I looked for my parking place? Did I drive right past them? Walk past some of them after I parked? I was frightened about gangs in cars, gangs with guns. If the SLA weren't already parked on that part of Benvenue Avenue, they were on the way.

Finally the three who had kidnapped Peter Benenson parked in the driveway of Patty Hearst's apartment. Armed with their automatic rifles and pistols, they went down the walkway between the apartment and the adjoining house that leads to the apartment entrance and knocked. When Patty's boyfriend, Steven Weed, opened the door, they rushed in, threw him to the floor, and began beating and kicking him. Patty Hearst was grabbed and carried screaming from the house. Weed finally managed to get loose and ran screaming from the apartment, while one of the men kept pointing his rifle at him with a cold smile on his face. A neighbor came to see what was happening: he was grabbed, beaten, and knocked unconscious to the floor, a floor that was already soaked with Steven Weed's blood. Two women who came out of the next apartment were driven back inside as automatic rifle fire splintered the shingled wall beside them. Patty's captors threw her in the trunk and fled in Peter Benenson's car, with Benenson still crouching terrified on the floor, expecting that the next shot would be for him. The two cars with the rest of the SLA roared away. The Patty Hearst story had begun.

Now I know that the only thing crazy about my experience was my insistence on thinking it was about my craziness. I was going into a potentially dangerous situation. There was a gang with guns who shot at people in the alleyways between the houses in that neighborhood, they did beat people unmercifully, lots of people were terrified. Part of my mind was telling me to get away. I misinterpreted it as my craziness. Luckily nothing worse happened to me or Terry than fright and shame.

I learned about how the mind can transcend ordinary limitations at a very deep level. It's not just an abstract idea. I've since applied my lesson in several minor happenings: when I've had a strong psychological reaction that doesn't make "sense," given my understanding of myself, I try to remember to look more carefully at the world around me. I haven't had to dodge any bullets, but I have looked and found other people under stress or needing help. Now I wonder how many other people are tuning into the world around them this way and unnecessarily suffering because they think it's their own craziness? What could we be like if we could understand and deliberately use this kind of psychic sensitivity?

Finding the True Self Onstage:
Dialogue with a Comedienne

Casey Fraser
Rob Marchesani

Poets, philosophers and seers have always concerned
themselves with the idea of a true self, and the betrayal of the self
has been a typical example of the unacceptable.

–D. W. Winnicott/*The Concept of the False Self*

CF: Most of my material, most of what I say on stage is never written down. The written script I work with is barely a skeleton of what I end up saying on stage. That seems to change nightly as well. I do try to write down what I found myself saying on stage in order to create new scripts every so often . . .

RM: I did not know that, though much of the material is consistent with your last performances. So you really are an improvisationist?

CF: I find it more exciting to keep things improvisational in this kind of format. It keeps me honest. It has taken a while to find the structure I feel it

Casey Fraser is an Emmy-nominated actress, writer, and comedienne. Her theatrical background began at the age of six touring the East Village and the Middle East with LaMama's *Fragments of a Greek Trilogy* directed by Andre Serban. She has worked in theater, film, and television, and her most recent venture was the one-woman show *Why We Don't Bomb the Amish.*

Rob Marchesani is a psychotherapist in private practice in New York City where he teaches "The Internet and the Hyper-Self" at The New School in Greenwich Village. In 1996 he appeared in the Beth B film *Visiting Desire*, a documentary on fantasy and sexual relations which entered the Toronto and Berlin film festivals after playing at Cinema Village. He holds a Masters from The New School and is co-editor of *The Psychotherapy Patient* series.

[Haworth co-indexing entry note]: "Finding the True Self Onstage: Dialogue with a Comedienne." Fraser, Casey, and Rob Marchesani. Co-published simultaneously in *The Psychotherapy Patient* (The Haworth Press, Inc.) Vol. 11, No. 3/4, 2001, pp. 187-196; and: *Frightful Stages: From the Primitive to the Therapeutic* (ed: Robert B. Marchesani, and E. Mark Stern) The Haworth Press, Inc., 2001, pp. 187-196. Single or multiple copies of this article are available for a fee from The Haworth Document Delivery Service [1-800-342-9678, 9:00 a.m. - 5:00 p.m. (EST). E-mail address: getinfo@haworthpressinc.com].

© 2001 by The Haworth Press, Inc. All rights reserved.

needs on top of which I can improvise. This current show has been more strict than I'd like it to become in its next incarnation. Does that make sense?

RM: I think so. In your last performance of *WHY WE DON'T BOMB THE AMISH,* there were moments when I thought, this is what therapy is all about. You were asking, "Isn't this what we all want?" Can you say more about this in terms of one's possible aims, purposes and/or search for meaning in life and psychotherapy?

CF: I guess it's hard for any performance not to feel a little like therapy in that both are on some basic level. True performance is a search for some kind of meaning. It bodes some understanding of why we all do what we do or feel what we feel. Whether very personal or very broad, a groping around for more clarity seems to me to be a constant. The broad sense of meaning sometimes turns out to feel personal. Yet this personal search ends up more universal and bigger than one would have originally thought. We are, after all, social creatures. We thrive within relationships affecting and being affected by each other, continually reminded moment to moment of our interdependency. We spend so much time needing to "stand out," to feel "unique." On some level I think we need to feel alike. Writers and performers of theater pieces are always creating a communal experience. We create a place to "search" together. One goes into therapy with a similar need: a search with someone else in order to confirm that "I am not standing alone."

RM: Can you imagine trembling as the manifestation of stage fright?

CF: Trembling in the literal, physical sense? Sure. I remember grade school plays. A child who would stand on the stage in front of the audience of parents, teachers and fellow students shaking uncontrollably while trying to deliver his lines. What a sad statue of vulnerability! Although that was never me. I experience stage fright in my own way, an inner trembling taking me from deathly fear as I face an audience. This trembling retrenches as energy with a sort of "life of its own." Here I am on stage "alone" with that audience.

RM: Now trembling, i.e., shivering, is a form of stage fright. Trembling when cold is the body's way of warming up. Is trembling before a performance a way of warming up to an audience?

CF: That's an interesting way of putting it. Yes, I think it is. Warming up to the audience is maybe just warming up to the idea of the audience or warming up to the performance itself. I don't think a performer can actually warm up to a specific audience until she meets them. Each audience is so unique and requires a unique relationship with the performer. In fact, I think for me, it's at the point where I finally meet my audience that the actual trembling stops and another energy moves into place.

RM: Assuming that stage fright may have positive effects on performance, have you discovered any way of maximizing its benefits?

CF: Trembling is something that happens alone once the audience becomes a part of the picture. Trembling is becoming one with another person's body heat. Then trembling can stop. At least that's what I experience. Even though an issue of sheer adrenaline, I'm nevertheless excited by the audience, its challenge, its danger. Such energy transforms from a shivering paralysis to a tremendous sense of strength.

RM: Does stage fright maximize (or cut one off from) an inner dialogue as one becomes established with the audience?

CF: Maximizing its benefits? Okay. Well, that's a tough challenge. I'm not sure I have a complete answer, but I do think that stage fright means that the performers really care about what they're doing. In and of itself, that's positive. Intense fear has the potential to be anything else intense. What counts is knowing how to guide it. I think stage fright can cut the performer off from the audience completely if the performer holds on like a security blanket. But there is also the potential to increase the bond between performer and audience. This happens if the fright is allowed to exist as a component in the "love" equation of performing. I love you therefore I am frightened to stand before you. Obviously, there needs to be trust as well as fear in that equation or yes, there is no communication and it remains uncomfortable for performer and audience alike. Doesn't love always come with fear?

RM: I think it does because love makes one naked in a very personal way. Few of us are so comfortable being naked.

CF: Being on stage is being naked in a way. I think a good performance makes the audience feel naked too. They need to feel vulnerable so that they too tremble. In the absence of unbared trembling, where's the catharsis? Stage fright should manifest into a mutual bond of love, hate, fear, or whatever between the performer and the audience. This again requires trust. But keep in mind that establishing the trust is initially in the hands of the performer. Performers have to be able to say, "Yes, I'm scared, but I care about you and I know what I'm doing here. So come along with me." In the absence of trembling, something is missing, forced, phony. An audience may be amused but never really drawn in by a performer without that element of vulnerability and truth. Stage fright ultimately maximizes the inner dialogue . . . but also always has the potential to overtake a performer, in an almost egotistical manner, and leave them cut off both from the audience as well as themselves. We're all scared when we get naked. If you aren't then you can't really care much about the situation.

RM: What is a director's role in stage fright?

CF: Primarily I think stage fright is very personal. It may even be embarrassing–so much so that it can be hidden by performers from fellow actors and directors. It is the director's role to be insightful enough to recognize the defense and help the performer shape the fear into something honest and useful on stage. The director's job is to recognize as much of what the performer has to offer as possible. Stage fright is part of that picture.

RM: You speak often about honesty. I can't help but think we are also dealing with opposing, dishonest forces. I wonder which are more threatening and which more freeing.

CF: What exactly do you mean by opposing dishonest forces?

RM: Well, maybe it is the "acting" when it is acting as opposed to just "being" on stage. I may also be thinking of characters who are dishonest in their roles. But more so, the reaching toward honesty. Do you come up against a kind of temptation to be dishonest? I wonder if stage fright is a battle for the "true" self to come forth.

CF: I'm a big believer in the "just being" onstage idea. That's the ultimate goal–to just be, but just be in a way that is so truthful that it cuts to a universal core, and is therefore inspired. That's not always easy. There is always a temptation to be dishonest. For some reason dishonesty can often feel like the safer choice, although the consequence is a horrible sense of emptiness and even guilt. I think there can be different kinds of stage fright. The battle for the true self to come forth is one and second there is the simple fear that nobody will like me. Although these two "frights" cross paths, one usually is the stronger force. I find that the fear that arises from that battle for the true self often is a direct result of the realization that the true self will not and cannot be liked by everyone.

RM: Is there an experience (something the opposite of stage fright) we might term as "great expectations" or performance awe?

CF: Sure. They are two sides of the same coin and often one does not come without the other. Performance awe is not a result of cockiness, thinking: "I'm really going to be great." I think it has more of an effect as a result of being affected by the power of the dialogue between performer and audience. This becomes the magical covenant they enter into together for the duration of the performance. I've always felt that theatres are very much like churches. It's that same power inherent in both that instills fear. There is an undeniable gravity to the situation even if in light comedy. Even light comedy can be inspired and fulfilling.

RM: Well, yes. It gives us permission or reminds us that we can laugh at ourselves.

CF: Clowns are very cathartic, and very scary too.

RM: Well, we have Steven King (*IT*) to thank for that.

CF: In a way. Although what's funny about them is the exaggeration of our own vulnerabilities. That's pretty scary when you come to think about it.

RM: Well, there you have the two faces of theater again. Do some actors, comedians, dancers use drugs or alcohol to enhance their performance? And, if so, what are the limitations inherent in such practices?

CF: I think so. The same way anybody uses these substances to feel better about life in general. And of course we're always looking for the power pill, the steroid that will make us the best at what we do. Performers are always looking to "get out of their heads" and "into the moment." Therefore, drugs and alcohol follow. Of course the pitfall is, I think, that the line becomes blurred as to when the substance is helping you get out of your head enough to be "spontaneous" and/or "inspired" and when that same chemical is just helping you forget how unspontaneous and uninspired you are.

RM: Does improvisation cause more or less stage fright?

CF: Do you mean improvisation? Or are you referring to the lead-in to training to the use of actual improvisation during a performance? I think the training is helpful in terms of learning to trust the fear enough to let it work good magic rather than bad on stage. In terms of using it in performance, I'm not sure about that. I tend to use it when I am performing my own work, but it's always something that just happens. Maybe an improvisation is part of the awe. In other words I don't think about it before I'm on, while I'm in the trembling pre-performance mode.

RM: Can psychotherapy help with stage fright? For example, some analysts feel that stage fright is an unanswered infantile appeal for mother's comfort.

CF: Can't good psychotherapy help with anything? The appeal for mother's comfort. Yeah, of course that's a part of it. I think a lot of life is "Mommy don't leave the room, I'm not asleep yet." That's the human experience which is universal. So I think that part of stage fright is good. It's real. It can reach an audience if channeled correctly.

RM: Maybe that's how good psychotherapy works. Facing life with a new confidence.

CF: Sounds right to me.

RM: I've often thought, fear isn't absent in our heroes, nor in our actors. It's just that heroes and actors make the decision to go forward anyway. To simply be. Stage anticipates what? Is it true that some actors experience numbness rather than performance anxiety?

CF: Confidence is very much about accepting and embracing our vulnerabilities and weaknesses. If we can do that we can also see our strengths in a new light. Without weaknesses there are no strengths. It's all about relationship. Oh yes, the greatest strength is always going on anyway. Numbness to me is the problem. It is like denial. But I don't know how other people process it. I guess it's possible to feel numb in preparation of feeling a tremendous amount all at once when the show begins.

RM: Some performers get anxious after a performance. Of these, some try to avoid any personal contact following their leaving the stage.

CF: I usually shy away from contact when I feel I haven't come through. I feel guilty and empty. But this again is such a personal thing.

RM: So there's a deflation if you weren't "on."

CF: And of course if you've really put yourself out there, there is always that residual effect, the need to "come down" and it often feels inappropriate to face people during that time. A deflation? Let me think. I wouldn't really put it that way, because I don't feel there is ever really an inflation. I think the image of the puffed up cockiness goes along with the kind of performing that prompts people to say, "I killed them." It's an ego thing, some sort of battle with winners and losers. I can't deal with performing like that. I think that's why comedy clubs so turned me off. It really all comes down to contact and honesty. If I feel I have not made contact with the audience, I do feel like I failed. That's the emptiness. The anxiety. The loneliness. And the questioning. Should I really be doing this? I think that's where performing differs from another profession that maybe is not so tied into a person's sense of self worth.

RM: Do audiences' responses abate and/or prolong stage fright? Do other performers?

CF: That's the constant battle. You can't deny the fact that we all affect each other. If audiences are unresponsive or negative one night, it is going to heighten the ongoing inner battle with the demons of worthiness. On the other hand, if they are exceptionally responsive and positive, it's more like having a great conversation. Maybe even a love affair. The energy feeds on itself and it's wonderful. Fear gives way to awe.

RM: Can you say more about that?

CF: Fear gives way to awe when the dialogue works. I truly think it is as simple as that. Communication is godly.

RM: Have you ever "whited out," forgotten your lines?

CF: Yes, I have gone blank on stage. That is the only time I can remember feeling numb. It's a situation that calls for a certain kind of adrenaline kicking in.

RM: There have been musicians who feel they're playing off-key–when they aren't, dancers who feel their bodies are out of synch–when the dance is actually well-executed, and actors who feel they've missed their persona–when they may have created an even more engaging character.

CF: That's true. We can be terrible self-judges. It's a fine line to walk, trying to communicate creation. I think it's the occasion when the audience and the performer are in synch with each other in an inspired and truthful way. Here the sense of awe is in play. I certainly don't feel it every time I'm on stage, and yet I have had "successful" shows as far as audiences are concerned. Doing something new and wonderful and feeling it was off is just an example of how much we have to learn about ourselves and how we will never be finished learning.

RM: Is it ever helpful to have a known friend or other ally in the audience?

CF: Sometimes yes, sometimes no. People you know come with their own baggage. I think it's best when it doesn't matter. No matter who is out there the show is about meeting people anew.

RM: Are there stages of stage fright?

CF: I think so, but I've never made a study of them. I know I can count on getting slightly queasy and anxious and having those emotions build to full-fledged terror. But then right before the show begins the feelings transform to a calmer state, though no less intense. Maybe it's a sort of resignation to the situation. Nowhere to run. Nowhere to hide. Sounds horrible, doesn't it? But I think it's all good. Then when I step on stage it's any number of feelings, because at that point it's no longer just about me.

RM: Were you a shy kid? Is shyness related to stage fright? Is it a throw-back?

CF: I was pretty shy. But I was also very talkative and pretty wild when I wanted to be. I'm not sure I can answer that question in any general way. I would think even people who were complete extroverts can experience stage fright. I don't really think it's a throwback. I think that would make it very stunting. I think it's something that is about the here and the now and dealing with it with all the unknowns involved. Of course there are parts of us that are always children and in that sense some of that fear and sense of insignificance of childhood is there.

RM: Is it possible that certain personas you adopt as an actor experience more/less stage fright than others?

CF: I think it is quite possible for some stage personas or characters to elicit more stage fright than others. My experience of stage fright is that it is truly an issue in the pre-show waiting phase. I think action sort of overrides stage fright. I don't think it's possible to be "in character" on stage while experiencing stage fright. Stage fright includes a sense of awareness of the "onstage" situation–something like, "Can I come through?" anxiety. When one is involved in the performance, other fears, fears more truthful to the character or onstage persona may exist or even come out of that initial stage fright. Nevertheless, actual performance fear is a fear of anticipation. So I guess what I'm getting at is the difference between a character "experiencing" stage fright versus the anticipation. Here the act of "getting into" character elicits more or less stage fright. This is not unlike other life situations. Anticipation, conquering anticipation, preparing . . . and finally making the leap into action are the most difficult moments to conquer.

RM: Getting back to psychotherapy as help or hindrance. Some analysts account for performance anxiety as energy blockages–a form of emotional or psychic resistance. Comment?

CF: The idea of performance anxiety as energy blockages poses an interesting dilemma in terms of how to deal with it. Sure, I think stage fright can block all kinds of positive creative things just as any intense anxiety in life can. Fear is debilitating. On the other hand, the stage fright itself is energy. And sometimes this type of energy, specifically when dealing with performance whether it's theatrical or other, is so concentrated into a specific moment that it acts like a rush intensifying that moment in preparation for the act to follow, as well as an indication that that moment is meaningful enough to command this kind of intense feeling. How wonderful it is to care this much about a moment in time, about one's contribution to that moment. Therefore I feel the best way to deal with stage fright is not to look at it as a block but rather as an energy, a gift, waiting to be utilized and focused in a positive way. Seeing it as the enemy, a negative personality quirk that must be overcome, is to strip it, and oneself, of a certain kind of power. Maybe that power has something to do with vulnerability and humanity and of feeling something, not just thinking something, but really feeling it throughout one's entire body and mind. To me that's what stage fright is, a forceful and powerful onslaught of feeling. It can feel bigger than oneself. I have learned from my own experiences to be more afraid of nonchalant pre-show feelings then of stage fright.

On the other hand, it is not all black and white and I think the final result of extreme stage fright often results in creative blockages, distorted ideas of self and a focus so set on, "Am I okay?" that there is no room to delve into character or theatrical revelation. At these times it is like being in a house of mirrors where everywhere you look you see YOU. Frightening and destructive. That's when it becomes paralyzing and acts like a complete and utter resistance to the situation at hand. In the end it's a matter of accepting, embracing stage fright, understanding the power of one's own sense of vulnerability and the energy that a rush of this kind of fear offers. And then the fright hits like a wave, using the fear by insisting on seeing beyond one's own ego, not getting caught in that house of mirrors.

RM: And then there are cognitive-behaviorists who feel that stage fright is phobic-like and with positive imagery and reassurance, can be reversed.

CF: See, I'm just not sure about the idea of reversal. I certainly feel that fear, any fear can be so debilitating that it becomes a phobia, but I also believe stage fright is such a natural part of performing that it can't and shouldn't be eliminated. It's not a disease. It's a human response to the responsibility and intensity of involving others in a very personal journey. Positive imagery or anything else that helps channel the fear or anxiety into a more positive energy is wonderful. I just feel that approaching stage fright as a "problem" that needs to be eliminated becomes a problem in itself. My fear is that becoming so obsessed with the fear and with the killing of the fear that I might inhibit my own emotions before a show.

RM: Then there are bioenergetic oriented therapists who see an inversion of self, where defensive muscular reactions become bodily blockages. In these cases, the actor literally ceases to breathe. Comment?

CF: I've never experienced this myself, although I have certainly experienced a feeling of not being able to take a deep breath, racing heart and other definite physical side effects of stage fright. The mind and the body are quite inseparable aren't they? Sometimes it's that physical sensation of butterflies or racing heart that comes on, almost out of the blue, forcing me to stop whatever else I am doing or thinking about and reminding me, "It's time to focus on your task at hand." In other words, the physical definitely precedes the mental process of preparing for the show. Again, I guess I am seeing this as a positive, necessary reaction to the process of preparing and performing. Yet not breathing sounds pretty scary. A little deathlike actually. Once in a while, usually when I'm in a pretty chaotic period of life, I find myself waking in a panic, feeling that I stopped breathing in my sleep, and gasping for air, breathing in as deeply as possible. So maybe this is a sort of shock to the system similar to the experience of stage fright. When you stop breathing you are forced to gasp deeply, fill your lungs as fast as you can with as much air as possible. It's a gut reaction. So if you are feeling uninspired, numb, unprepared, whatever the case might be, this could act as just the kick-start needed to plunge into the focus and energy needed to perform.

RM: A patient reported to her therapist that the closest image that comes to her when she experiences stage fright is a fantasy of wanting to run away from a rapist–except she feels paralyzed by terror. Another patient, also an actress, found great relief of performance anxiety by carrying a pack of cigarettes, viewing them as her reward for a good performance. A man suffered so from stage fright and particularly audition anxiety. He "solved" his problem by doing children's theatre and performing in front of children in pediatric wards in city hospitals. Comment on any or all of these?

CF: Well, wanting to run away but feeling paralyzed I think is a pretty common event. The specific image of the rapist certainly makes sense considering the idea of becoming "naked" in front of the audience. The question remains: Does the rapist represent the audience or herself? After all, performing is not a sentence, it is (99% of the time) a choice. So, is she afraid that she is going to rape herself by submitting herself to the performance? I guess in a sense she is. There is always a little self-betrayal when one puts oneself out in front of others in such a personal way. We are constantly betraying ourselves (or at least our image of ourselves) when we invite others in. Just like any relationship. There is always betrayal, just as there must be trust. And between the two, I think, comes the exciting walk on the tightrope of human-to-human contact.

The Little Old Lady

Pietro Arpesella

SUMMARY. Stage fright often affects the body as well as the mind. A stage requires a body to be present and that body has its own reactions to the emotions that are stirred by the person's thoughts. In the following article, a swell of panic brings one performer's childhood experience of family and self into a battle with diabetes and its causes.

KEYWORDS. Cause-effect, diabetes, femininity, cancer, childhood, anger, hysteria, impulses

---

After being a successful investment banker, Pietro Arpesella became an actor and writer and took his craft from Italy to New York City. He has worked extensively as an actor in Italy and in independent movies and Off-Broadway shows in New York. Recently, he gave the voice to three characters in the English version of *Life Is Beautiful*, and you can hear him in the "Mike's Best Friend's Boyfriend" episode of *Spin City* as the "Roberto NO!" guy. In July he guest starred on two episodes of Italy's number one soap, *Vivere*. He recently completed a role as the host of Cult Network Italia, and appeared in the new Canal+ movie *Business Sense*.

Arpesella wrote, directed and performed a one-man show called *Life & Me . . . What A Couple!* which has just completed two highly successful runs in New York City and Pittsburgh. His first screenplay is currently under consideration by major studios in both New York and Los Angeles, and *Run with Me*, another screenplay of his, just won the Special Jury Prize at the screenplay competition of the New York International Film & Video Festival, 2000. He has recently begun writing *Living in America*, a TV comedy show, which is getting attention in the industry. He performed an excerpt from *Living in America* at the Cornelia Street Cafe, Greenwich Village, NY, which received thriving enthusiasm and appreciation from audience and industry.

Address correspondence to: Pietro Arpesella (E-mail: Pietro33@aol.com).

[Haworth co-indexing entry note]: "The Little Old Lady." Arpesella, Pietro. Co-published simultaneously in *The Psychotherapy Patient* (The Haworth Press, Inc.) Vol. 11, No. 3/4, 2001, pp. 197-203; and: *Frightful Stages: From the Primitive to the Therapeutic* (ed: Robert B. Marchesani, and E. Mark Stern) The Haworth Press, Inc., 2001, pp. 197-203.

It's Sunday, early afternoon. I just went over the new material I am about to perform, but I keep having this feeling: "Something is going to happen." I approach the small stage and I see a couple of sweet old ladies that had seen my show two nights before and said they would come to see me today at the Italian Festival, in downtown Pittsburgh, Pennsylvania. Sara, my publicist, is running around trying to find out if there is a microphone or even just anybody to talk to. I hang out with the ladies for some casual chit chatting.

They are sweet. I am happy they are here today to see me again. Yet, I look around, distancing myself from what the ladies are saying, and I don't get any feeling that a show is about to begin on that stage, let alone my show.

Sara approaches fast and says, "I talked to the guy, he said you can perform on the main stage in the main square. Let's go."

The "guy" welcomes me and explains that apparently the people in charge of the small stage must have had something going on because they didn't show up. I can perform at 2:00 p.m., on the main stage. I say, "Great." He tells me, "The only thing is that the orchestra will be setting up while you are performing." I say, "That's fine." We shake hands and he goes away. I think, "This is going to be interesting."

Sara and I sit at a table waiting for two o'clock. On the stage an Italian woman is playing her classical guitar. There are a few people scattered in the few hundred chairs. I suddenly feel I am not really present and something is going on but I don't know what it is and I am just acting okay on the outside.

Sara asks me if I feel that a disease has a relationship to how we respond to life. I say, "Of course. Nothing happens by chance, it is always a cause-effect type relationship. Even when we can't explain something, there is always a cause that generated it. We might not be able to identify or understand the cause rationally, but that doesn't qualify things as casualties. It's just that we don't see the action-reaction chain of events." Sara asks me, "Do you feel the same with respect to cancer?" I say, "I feel the same about everything. In some cases the cause effect relationship is very complex and difficult to understand. If you punch me in the face, I get a blue eye. That's simple to understand. If a girl grows up in a family that doesn't validate her femininity and imposes a sense of 'wrong-being' and guilt on her, once a woman she is likely to develop breast cancer, or ovarian cancer, depending on the type of issues she has, like my mother did. In this case the cause-effect relationship is more compounded and could be difficult to grasp."

Take me, for example. I got diabetes when I was six years old and my parents were fighting badly and finally separated. I felt an incredible pressure and pain, which I couldn't turn into anger, because I had to be the perfect kid/friend/man for my mother, the perfect brother/father/friend for my sister, and I couldn't risk turning away any further my already absent father, because I desperately needed him to give me a sense of my male self.

Although all the elements were there, I couldn't get crazy and become a psychotic kid, because that would have meant losing my mother forever, because she wanted a perfect kid, one that she could be proud of and use to validate the motherly side of her femininity. So my brain had to function. But in that situation, which was severely lacking in sweetness for me, I felt something was very wrong with me and my ability to receive the sweetness of life, which is love. My mother was giving it to me only if I satisfied her requests, and it wasn't really love, it was more like "attention" or a "Good, now do this other thing for me" type of thing. My father was gone and I felt he was jealous of me because of how my mother was with me.

Maybe I didn't even like my father that much, but he was the only alternative to my mother and I felt very guilty for feeling that. So I felt I was a really bad kid, who actually didn't even have the right to exist, and they were actually doing me a favor by enduring my presence. I couldn't get that sweetness of life, that love that changes the chemical composition of the blood and makes it sweeter, more yin. So, I got diabetes. I copped out and "decided," on a subconscious level, to redirect and internalize all the pain of not getting the love that I needed to feel entitled to exist.

The resulting anger that I couldn't express on the outside, I blocked it into the pancreas, the organ that regulates the degree of sweetness of our blood. I had my immune system attack the islet of Langerhans in the pancreas and stop them from producing insulin so that my blood would have a "sweeter" chemical composition, resembling that of someone when he/she is loved. I got diabetes. Now, on the outside, I still was the perfect kid, so Mom would be happy. My brain was functioning so I could be the first in class. But, I was also sick. This meant Daddy had to take care of me and could treat me with gentleness and sweetness, without running the risk of being "too feminine" or "not cool for a boy," and, who knows, maybe now that I was sick, my parents might even get back together.

"If you're ready you can go," the guy says to me. "Do you mind introducing yourself?" I say, "Of course not," and I am on stage. It is a large stage, maybe six feet above the ground, and in front of me is the entire square with innumerable rows of empty chairs, with only a few people scattered here and there. In the second row there is a family, mother, father and two kids. The mother is looking at me, and that makes me feel good.

I start warming up the audience as my voice runs through the microphone to all corners of the square. But there is a strange feeling because I don't really hear myself. The place is huge, and I get a feeling of distance from the audience which I don't like. I start talking about the fact that I'd just gotten a driver's license in New York and how that was quite an experience, very different from when I got a driver's license in Italy.

As I am going through the material somebody is listening, somebody else isn't and I can see them because we are in full daylight. I talk about how in the Five-Hour Class you take in New York all they really talk about is drunk driving and that you shouldn't drink and drive. "If you don't drink and you never drove before, they should really have you take the Five-Minute Class, because at the end of the Five-Hour Class all you know is that you shouldn't drink and drive, which doesn't really make a difference to you because you didn't drink in the first place. You also learn that you shouldn't drive faster than 55 mph, but you have absolutely no idea how to get to 55 mph."

Then I glance at the husband of the family sitting in front of me, and he has become totally numb and stares ahead to the empty space. I think, "I bet he knows something about drunk driving." I keep going, but I feel, "This is not the right material for this audience."

All of a sudden I hear "WWWHHOOO, WHHEEE." I look down and at the foot of the stage is a full orchestra warming up and tuning the instruments. I think "This is interesting" and I keep going, although I see that even the mother now isn't really having fun. Then I look over to my left and I see a little old lady waving her arm way up in the air. And I think, "Is she waving at me? It can't be. . . . Is she waving at me?"

Something happened to me in that moment. It was as if there was one me working on the piece talking about the driver's license, and basketball, baseball, football, and another me watching the first me. I was seeing myself with the microphone in my face, a seemingly fun face but with a strong layer of tension underneath my skin. My body, loaded with the pressure of inappropriate material for the type of crowd, was talking and moving on stage, and still the little old lady kept waving in my direction. "What is she doing?" I keep thinking. "Is she waving at me?"

"WWWHHHOOO, WWWHHEE. . . ." The orchestra and the instruments get louder and louder. Now the me that is speaking the words of the piece is holding on to that piece of material for sheer life, like a shipwrecked person would hold on to a floating log. I know I am pushing it, yet I hold on to it as if I have no other choice.

Silently, inside myself I think, "I am starting to panic." On the outside it doesn't show, because I am going on and I am almost done. Just one more line to go, but inside I am freaking out. Suddenly, I feel that everybody else wants me out of there. The orchestra is purposely louder and louder to cover up the crap that I'm uttering from my mouth. But instead of reacting to all those external stimuli, I feel like I am caged inside my body and I am imploding. I glance down and the little old lady is now standing there by the first row. She is waving and she yells straight to my face, "DON'T YOU SEE? NOBODY IS LISTENING TO YOU!"

Then all was silent and still, like in a snapshot. The orchestra was silent and not moving, the people were motionless in front of me and the little old lady was frozen with her hand up in the air waving at me. For a split second, which inside of me lasted for a defined eternity, the air choked in my throat, my brain went blank with no oxygen to feed it, and I felt I wasn't supposed to be there, I wasn't entitled to be there. I felt I was an unnecessary piece of meat that everybody had to put up with. In that split second I felt a change happening inside of me, I became hysterical, actually I became a hysterical woman. I dropped the last line of the piece and, coming out of that frozen eternity, I said, "Well, I seem to have offended somebody here, so I'm gonna stop, the orchestra is almost ready. You have been great. Come see my show tonight . . ." and I invited everybody to the closing night of my show in town.

I walked off that stage and I was feeling this rigid thing inside of me, where the solar plexus is, as if something had become thick and hard. Sara was looking at me, speechless. One of the sweet ladies quickly approached and said, "You shouldn't have left, she"–referring to the little old lady–"is a little crazy you know." I said that it was okay, and thank you for being there. We said good-bye and Sara and I started to walk toward the car.

I kept walking fast and talking out loud. Sara was following me. I was walking so fast it was clear I was running away from something very painful, an old feeling, the feeling of not being entitled to exist. But where was I running? Nowhere, really. Or maybe yes, I was running to myself, but I didn't know it yet.

The first thing I felt was that I was angry at myself, for the way I reacted at the whole situation–like when I was a kid and my parents were distant and unavailable, I thought there was something wrong with me. That was my first professional flop. Yet, I was feeling that something really good had just happened to me. I sure didn't know what it was yet, because it really felt like shit, but something good had just happened. In my mind I started picturing all the things I could have done different.

First of all, I could have used different material, but I didn't really have it, so I couldn't have done that. I could have walked up to the little old lady, I could have shaken her hand and said, "Thank you for being an ass," and walked away. Yes, I would have liked to have done that, very much. Very dramatic, but I didn't do that either.

We had a few hours before we had to be at the theater for the show, so Sara drove me around for a while and waited for me to calm down. We agreed on the fact that it wasn't the right material for the setting and the type of audience. But while we were talking I said, "You see, I saw a woman telling me that I wasn't desired, and I freaked. I didn't use it, or respond to it, or even ignore it. I just felt she was right and I freaked. This is why I still have diabetes." And then I started to feel what had actually just happened.

All those feelings I had, the feeling that something had hardened where the solar plexus is, that's where the pancreas is. In fact, as I was telling Sara before I went on stage, my pancreas hardened when I was a kid, it became still because back then, as I just did now, I had the feeling that I wasn't desired, that I wasn't entitled to exist, and I felt it was my fault and I had to go away. All the anger and every impulse I felt toward the outside world, I redirected it internally and choked my own being in the pancreas. In fact, the name pancreas comes from the ancient Greek and means "all flesh." I choked myself in the organ that represents my being in the flesh, my being in the body, my existing on this earth. In killing the Langerhans cells that produce insulin, I symbolically and physically killed my existence in this body on this earth.

Furthermore, on that stage, I realized that I had relived another very crucial moment of my life directly connected to the cause-effect chain of events that resulted in me getting diabetes–my birth. I had a great and beautiful nine months inside my mother's womb. When I felt it was time for me to get out and bring all that beauty and good feelings to the next level of existence, the earth level, I found myself upside down and had a breach birth. The umbilical cord was wrapped around my throat so tight I almost died, if it weren't for the doctor who cut the cord at the last second when I was completely cyanotic. So the message I got there from my mother, who at that moment was the entire universe for me, was "You are not welcome here on this earth. It was good while you were inside, but you shouldn't have desired to come out, your impulse is not good. In fact, when you follow your impulse, you die (the choking)."

So when my parents were fighting and all that tension and pain was in the air, and I would have wanted to yell and scream and do something so that they understood that it was bad and I wanted something different, I didn't follow those impulses, because I had been taught at birth that, "My impulses are bad. I am unwanted, not entitled to be here." When I was six, I redirected all those impulses internally rather than express them and in so doing, locked them into the pancreas. Now, while I was on stage and everything froze on me, in that second, I choked. I actually felt my throat strangled and no oxygen going to my brain. I had just relived the two mechanisms that eventually caused me to have diabetes. That has got to be a good thing. So I started to be very grateful to the little old lady and her being an ass. First of all, she actually spoke the truth. I mean, couldn't I see that nobody was listening to me? Yes, I did see it, but what did I do? Nothing, I held on to the piece and pushed through it. And then she allowed me to relive a very crucial chain of events. This time around, I still behaved in the same way as I did when I was a child, and I redirected all the impulses internally instead of using them and adjusting to them. I still felt I wasn't entitled to be there, I was an unwanted piece of flesh. But at least, this time around, I became aware of the mechanism, and that is really good.

A half-hour before curtain that evening at the theater, I was still processing the events of the afternoon. I kept thinking, "It'll be interesting to see what will happen to me tonight on stage." Sara came to the dressing room. "Ten minutes," she said. "You know," I said, "As soon as I felt I didn't really have the audience with me, I should have ended at any reasonable point in the material, and on a light note thanked and invited everybody to the show tonight." Sara agreed, and we laughed thinking how much better it was that it happened there than on Broadway. "One minute. . . . Thirty seconds . . ." and, it is show time. That night I performed the best show of the entire run, and I felt very good. I allowed myself to be extremely visible and vulnerable on stage. I felt that every cell in my body had the right to exist, and it felt good.

Since I started working on myself and listening to my soul and my body, my health and diabetic condition have significantly improved. I now take a low amount of insulin which has been following a decreasing trend. Six years ago my eyes had the first signs of retinopathy, one of the diabetic complications. Today I have twenty-twenty vision, the retina has completely healed, and my general test results show a normal person in good health. Among other things that I do to improve my health, I am working with a therapist who has worked with another twenty-five-some-year type one diabetic woman who completely healed from diabetes and now lives free of any medication with a fully functioning pancreas. He is looking forward to when I will test negative to include my story in his book.

I am in the healing process and the most important thing is that I take care of myself. When this story took place, I did reenact the behavior that mirrored my getting diabetes, which means I am not free of it yet, of the causes. But I became aware of them, I relived them and felt it happening at a conscious level, and awareness definitely is a good step. Oftentimes angels come dressed up in funny ways, and they have to act like an ass or we might not even see them. Thank you, little old lady.

Poetic Schizophrenia:
Regarding the Performative Process
of Composition

John Schertzer

SUMMARY. Colonized by language, the body becomes written over and familiarized, possessed by the ego. When one pays attention to what is not yet familiarized, part of oneself becomes "other-ized," causing dread. Hence, the "performance anxiety." One feels invaded and feels the need to take possession. Writing schizophrenically is a way of exploring the unknown, the gaps between body and its impulses, and definition in an attempt to sketch a map without the usual epistemological systems possessing the ground. A free-play form of experimentation tends to take place more often in poetry than in narrative or expository prose, simply because it is often its own subject, as well as proceeding closer to primary processes. John Ashbery is an example of a poet who writes–in his words–from free association, while Michael Palmer seems to engage the network of signifiers more purposefully. Both explore the points at which language and identity dismantle each other in an attempt to open further ground. *[Article copies available for a fee from The Haworth Document Delivery Service: 1-800-342-9678. E-mail address: <getinfo@ haworthpressinc.com> Website: <http://www.HaworthPress.com> © 2001 by The Haworth Press, Inc. All rights reserved.]*

KEYWORDS. Literature, performance anxiety, stage fright, signifiers, polyvocality, splintering, dissociation, fragmentation, language, metaphor, self-composition

---

John Schertzer teaches poetry at The New School in New York City, and is an editor of *LIT*.

[Haworth co-indexing entry note]: "Poetic Schizophrenia: Regarding the Performance Process of Composition." Schertzer, John. Co-published simultaneously in *The Psychotherapy Patient* (The Haworth Press, Inc.) Vol. 11, No. 3/4, 2001, pp. 205-221; and: *Frightful Stages: From the Primitive to the Therapeutic* (ed: Robert B. Marchesani, and E. Mark Stern) The Haworth Press, Inc., 2001, pp. 205-221. Single or multiple copies of this article are available for a fee from The Haworth Document Delivery Service [1-800-342-9678, 9:00 a.m. - 5:00 p.m. (EST). E-mail address: getinfo@haworthpressinc.com].

There has always been much mystique about madness. Saints of all faiths, as well as the most visionary of artists, and even scientists–Freud and Jung not excluded–have been considered so, particularly during their own lifetimes, and there has always been an apparent correlation between creative genius and madness. Then there are the so-called *anti-intellectual* intellectuals, such as Nietzsche, who insisted that things such as intuition, even superstition, both faculties of unreason, are requisite components of reason.[1] Though this comes as no surprise to us now, it has taken a paradigm shift for western civilization to accept in a serious light. It is no longer unusual for scientists, and even those arch-logicians, the mathematicians, to speak of intuitive leaps through which they make their discoveries.

This is only important to us because of how it has helped to redefine reality and unreality, sanity and insanity, as well as what is reasonably considered self and non-self. Social scientists have given us new ways of thinking about sanity; hence the border between normal and abnormal has become increasingly difficult to locate, or even imagine. Literature has found this environment a fertile soil, and quite haphazardly many writers have constructed alternatives to the traditional unified speaker who addresses the reader as a consistent and authoritative voice, as well as new paradigms with which to study their own subjectivity. This trend also corresponds to the tendency for artists to work in non-representational forms, those who no longer desired their work to be a portrayal of nature, since the artist herself is *nature*.[2] Since it has become almost commonplace to see the *actual* world as a thing dependent on an often unreliable observing-defining self, it has become more interesting for many artists to chart the progress of their own minds, rather than to strike truths like colonizing banners into an objective world which may not even exist.

Ironically enough, the skill perhaps most important to a poet, any artist whatsoever, the ability to transform the abstract into the concrete, is also a chief symptom of schizophrenia, surely what makes a schizo a schizo.[3] Central to any delusional system is the mechanism which transforms an abstraction into metaphor or simile, and then into a misjudgment of reality. The well-adjusted person may say something like, "She is poisoning my life," referring to how he or she is affected by another person, through the *toxic* patterns of their interactions. The schizophrenic, confusing abstract and concrete processes, may actually believe that the other is administering harmful chemicals or substances. These substances may have lethal physical effects, but they may also be the embodiment of spiritual illness as well.[4] Silvano Altieri calls this a "collapse of the abstract function into the concrete," and says that there is often a period of time in which many soon-to-be full-blown schizos can discern the difference between both thought processes, have access to both, and can move fluidly between one and the other. His question is: what is it that makes the schizophrenic lose his ability to make this distinction, his ability to *test reality*?[5] For it is perhaps a preferred state, this place in between, where the person can still distinguish between fact and falsity, while having access to a robust, magical world of metaphorical signification. This is perhaps the ideal of the poet, part of what he works at developing in himself. And while it is not looked at in specifically such a way by the theoreticians, Gilles Deleuze and Felix Guatarri, it is a subject they spin around in much of their two volumes of *Capitalism and Schizophrenia: Anti-Oedipus* and *A Thousand Plateaus*.[6]

To Deleuze and Guatarri the world of a schizophrenic is one where the distinctions between *man* and *nature* break down, as well as the distinctions between *producing* and *consuming*. The schizophrenic no longer experiences life in dichotomies, but in a way in which every consumption produces something, and every production consumes, as a process of *desiring-production*. From this vantage point it is no longer necessary, or even possible, for the ego to stand aside and forge representations of nature, since nature is ever-producing itself through infinite processes, where *subject* and *object* collapse into a generalized pool of *producer-product*. This may have been what Jackson Pollock meant when he said, "I am nature," seeing himself as one link in an endless chain, not the self-appointed nature deity some may have assumed he meant.

The work of poets like John Ashbery may be best understood in this light. Until one is used to his way of writing, many of his poems do in fact seem like schizophrenic babble. The disruptions of sense in his "How Much Longer Will I Be Able to Inhabit the Divine Sepulcher . . ."[7] clearly illustrate this:

> How much longer will I be able to inhabit the divine sepulcher
> Of life, my great love? Do dolphins plunge bottomward
> To find the light? Or is it rock
> That is searched? Unrelentingly? Huh. And if some day
>
> Men with orange shovels come to break open the rock
> Which encases me, what about the light that comes in then?
> What about the smell of the light?
> What about the moss?

These first two stanzas can easily be taken for the splintered rantings of a disorganized mind, not only because of the juxtaposition of unrelated or contradictory ideas, but also because of the unusual rhythmic patterns engendered in the lines, a nervous sputtering which accents the disruptions of logic. Just as Pollock's drip paintings may have seemed like mere random splatterings of paint, Ashbery's language seems to fall together in unrelated fragments. Perhaps it is even stranger for someone to use words in such a way, since paint might splatter haphazardly on its own, but words are generally willed together in such a way as to say something, if only out of habit. One might look at these stanzas and either imagine the speaker is speaking in a hermetic code, or that he is delusional in his feeling that he is communicating anything. Ashbery has thrown the power and authority of public discourse out the window. His writing is as non-rhetorical and non-didactic as possible. There may in fact be an aversion to didacticism at work here, something many of his disciples never took to heart. What is meant by a "divine sepulcher/Of life," for instance, and why is that followed by the "dolphins [which] plunge bottomward/To find the light"? He flees and thumbs his nose at authoritarian writing. In his defiance, as well as his sheer delight in strangeness and surprise, he smashes image, referent and qualifier together like rocks, follows one idea to the next in a narrative that is so unruly that it appears not to exist. And perhaps it doesn't.

But Ashbery's evasion of an authorial position doesn't result in his saying or teaching nothing. His work is an extreme version of *mind in action*, in which the object of meditation has become the imagination set loose from the constraints of the external world. It is, in some ways, a free-floating exploration of what Lacan termed *the network of signifiers*[7] which make up the "language" of the unconscious, similar to the work of the French Surrealists. This may be why the thought process resembles that of the dissociated schizophrenic, though it is intrinsically different. There may have been a choice, at some point, for the schizophrenic to dissociate himself from reality, though once that choice is made the break is complete. Ashbery's work results in the choice being made continuously. It is not madness, but a highly personalized style of thinking he has developed. It is the capacity for "distorted" thinking, and not the incapacity to be otherwise. *Reasonable behavior* is intrinsically public, impersonal, and authoritative, an array of roles taken on by mimicking the models we are given, those supposedly based on sets of rules and principles we tend to value. In this way we can survive in a world in which everyone is doing more or less the same thing. The same rules apply to literature, more or less, where physical survival is not as much a motive, but acceptance by a public audience is. Ashbery realizes that the "unified" speaker is a form of artifice, or performance, which may at times be the result of social pressures, or the anxiety of revealing oneself in ways that are not transparent to the reader, and a reader who is always primarily the "author." Much work goes into the guise of eloquence and authority, not only to block up any leaks of one's veiled core, but because of the monster one may create while one is not paying attention to the tacit details. Rejecting this model of voice construction makes for its own challenges, which we will see later.

Eloquence has always been highly valued in all literatures, but just as the camera had all but usurped the rights to landscape and portraiture, the proliferation of international-scale journalism and advertising has rendered such language impersonal. Some will even attach a political agenda to the habitual phraseology of our "common speech," since they see it as indicative of certain types of consumer behavior, both as a coddling of the marketplace, and as a consumption of ideology.[9] For them the masters of eloquence are the servants of corporate and political power, since no matter whose side you argue it's the actual structure of sense that has been bought and sold. Ashbery counters this situation by absorbing the rhetoric, and rearranging it with his own personal logic. For him it's not a matter of politics, but of personal freedom, and to use that freedom to be what he is, as he knows himself, at least on some level, not as a single, unified self, but as a polyphony of voices, desires and moods.

Gertrude Stein discussed the dubious relationship between personal language and public discourse, as far back as the nineteen-thirties, in *Everybody's Autobiography*, and perhaps even earlier. She certainly chose to write in the archly stylistic mode at least partially because of this relationship. It was no longer possible to write as people speak "because everybody talks as the newspapers and movies and radios tell them to talk the spoken language is no longer interesting and so gradually the written language says something and says it differently than the spoken language."[10] She goes on to say that everyday speech is the least personal of all types of language because of this, and that writing that seems overly stylistic and artificial is, in fact, more natural and personal. Nearly half a century later, Robert Grenier issued his proclamation "I HATE SPEECH," arguing that "all speeches say the same thing," as well as saying, "what now I want, at least, is the word way back in the head that is the thought or feeling forming out of the 'vast' silence/noise of consciousness experiencing the world *all the time*."[11] Though he was writing what was to be the beginning of *language poetry* poetics,[12] whose work was he better describing than Ashbery's, who not only avoids any connection with discourse, in most of his writing, but also writes in such a way as to insure itself against absorption in public speech, as it would be rather impossible to make use of it that way.

There is a familiarity to everyday talk and public discourse, one we take for granted, which is yet quite arbitrary, making all other forms of verbal communication seem strange, even pathological. Again, it is a *performance*. While many poets have used a more public mode of communication quite successfully, with undoubted originality, there are a number whose work has strayed from that tradition, identifying themselves more with what Grenier calls *the word in the back of the head* school of poetics. Whether they are aware of it or not, this takes into account a much different definition of *self*, one no longer identified with the circus ringmaster, but with the clowns, acrobats and animals. In simple terms, the *ego,* or conscious self, is created by the dialectic between the id (unconscious desire) and the superego (unconscious police force and board of editors), as it engages with the actual world. It is no more the *real* self than this paragraph is the actual stream of thoughts that passed through my head while I was writing it. Because, historically speaking, art often moves in more or less the same direction as does scientific and philosophical theory, and because parts of both eventually filter into the pool of popular wisdom, there is a continual evolution of self-definition, or definition of subjectivity. It has therefore become more acceptable, even ordinary, for people to identify themselves with their unconscious minds and its products: interpreting dreams, speaking of *Freudian slips* of the tongue, not to mention the proliferation of people actually in psychotherapy.[13] Moving backward from the comfortable and familiar terrain of the ego, one begins to penetrate the ever-strange world where unreason rules, and the self sounds more like a chorus than a solo singer, one of strange harmonies as well as discord, sometimes singing in concert, though often disrupting each other's song. This protean quality of the psyche we will refer to as polyvocality, a term I borrow from Deleuze and Guatarri, who have gone to great length to make us aware of how all things, ourselves most of all, are made up of an infinite array of meanings and forces.[14]

It is this constant disruption of the many voices engendered in John Ashbery's work that gives it its surface and rhythmical complexity. He ceases to pour his thoughts through the linearizing and legitimatizing funnel of his ego, and instead pushes everything forward against the window of the page, so that we experience the knots and coils–or *condensation*–of his thought process, instead of simply the result. This is the *network of signifiers* talking among themselves, perhaps magnetized by associative connections, a kind of *free association,* as he himself has described it. The "divine sepulcher/Of life" is a quick shift from one thing to its opposite, a disruption causing a complete change of direction, followed by "my great love," a phrase whose qualification ambiguously splits between both *sepulcher* and *life.* Next we are asked if "dolphins plunge bottomward/To find the light?" Surely, this is an absurd question, as is "Or is it rock/That is searched?" It is useful to look at the line endings, to see how quickly and radically every statement changes directions. There is a huge conceptual leap between *sepulcher* and *dolphin,* but at least dolphins can be said to *plunge bottomward* at times–but *To find the light?* The second half of the question completely disrupts our expectation, since it is rare that you would consider plunging downward beneath the surface to find light, at least in the physical sense of the word. But this notion of *light* relates back to the religiosity of the *divine,* and so is the idea of *plunging* beneath the surface. When he says "Or is it rock" we might think that it is not *light* the dolphins search for, but something tangible on the bottom, which would make more sense, until KA-BLAM! we feel our heads smash into that rock on the next line–"That is searched"–where we wonder if those dolphins actually dive into rock to search for light, which may be the flash that goes through one's head when it is struck hard. Each sign yields multiple possibilities and meanings, and the poem shows the numerous directions Ashbery's mind goes in as each arises, yielding next and its group of possibilities, splintering endlessly.

As the poem continues to develop the disruptions grow even more alarming. In the third stanza, following a brief description of what existence under the ground might be like, comes:

> I mean it–because I am one of the few
> To have held my breath under the house. I'll trade
> One red sucker for two blue ones. I'm
> Named Tom . . .

A relationship has already been set up between lying beneath the rocks, and swimming under water, so there is a reasonable connection to having *held my breath*, but the next sentence seems completely out of place, something a child would say to another child in an exchange of marbles or candy. The transition takes us in because the line break takes place after the subject and verb clause. To follow *I am one of the few . . . under the house* with *I'll trade* seems sensible, since the speaker seems to have something he'd like to trade, a mode of existence, for instance. But something quite unexpected follows in the next line. It's as if the speaker had begun one idea, and confused it with something completely incongruent, out of a loss of memory, or because of a stronger impulse driven to the surface.

There are plenty of breaks like this throughout the poem, a patchwork of discontinuities which begin to form a continuity of their own. The second line of the seventh stanza begins "And the reader is carried away/By a great shadow under the sea." At this point we can understand the connection between the *reader* being *carried away*, and the *steering wheel* of the next line, since they both involve modes of travel. But in the leap between the seventh and eighth stanzas something occurs which changes the direction of the sentence begun at the end of the seventh: "Behind the steering wheel// The boy took out his own forehead." In this case, the disruption in continuity is echoed by the disruption of travel, since there seems to have been a car crash in which *the boy* has injured his head. That "His girlfriend's head was a green bag/Of narcissus flowers" seems to suggest that she may have lost hers. This is of course not the only reading one might make of this section. Ashbery seems to have been telling us all along that everything in this poem can take off in different directions, as it has risen not out of a single source, but out of a confluence of impressions. In this way his work escapes paraphrase, since it is about a crisscrossing of ideas and energies, disjunctions and conjunctions of multiple voices.

Let's take a moment to consider a poem, this poem in particular, to be a "body, an endless weaving together of singular states, each of which is an integration of one or more impulses."[15] This is Brian Massumi's take on Deleuze's and Guattari's view of what it means to be a living entity. Each *state* may be seen as an idea, impression, gesture, habit, tick, which makes up an entire person. It does not matter that Ashbery didn't have access to this theoretical model when he wrote this poem. He intuited something similar in himself, his friends and acquaintances, and decided to play it out on the page, rather than lecture about it. The multiple voices in the piece may be different, but are all from the same source, something like the babbling of voices a schizophrenic may hear in moments of extreme dissociation, each rising out of a *singular state* or impulse. Ashbery has the uncanny ability to experience himself as a multiple whole, and not simply one piece at a time. This is not especially the experience of a novelist or playwright, who divvies himself up into a number of characters, all of which get to speak their minds, if not in complete sentences, then complete ideas. In such a case, the author is only changing masks, as well as voices, to create the illusion of there being more than one person in the room. Ashbery's experience is closer to what might be referred to as *egolessness*, since the ego might be looked at as a predominance of one state, or group of impulses.

"How Much Longer Will I Be Able to Inhabit the Divine Sepulcher" is like a launching pad from which many of Ashbery's later and much more complex poems take off, such as "Europe," "The Skaters," "The System," "A Wave," and the book-length *Flow Chart*. In these more sprawling projects the fragments tend to be longer and more luxurious, not as clipped and frenetic as those in the earlier poem. Their connections are also smoother and cloud-like, not the sharp, sudden shards we looked at previously. "The Skaters," for instance, is written in multiple voices, but each voice dominates a fairly long section, often lasting for pages. The transitions are much smoother as well, and rarely do we skip from one to another mid-sentence as in the previous example.

What is peculiarly interesting about "The Skaters" in particular is how Ashbery begins by piecing together something similar to the theoretical model of the body developed by Deleuze and Guattari, and it is therefore a good example of the art/theory parallel I mentioned above. D&G's version of *The Body* doesn't represent the flesh and blood body (although it can), but an abstract model of being, made up of multiple *states* or *planes of consistency*. In simple terms, each of these states can be looked at as one of the many personifications, or fragments of personifications which make up the entire person. Each state is called an *organ*, a single machine which links up with other machines, making a meta-machine whose existence is the sum of junctions and disjunctions, confluences and contradictions, congruent and conflicting desires. The self as such is in a state of chaos, often even at war with itself. No longer do we witness the performance anxiety of "getting it right," but a more basic form, as the fear of exposure becomes a dominant guiding principle in the overall shaping of the composition. There is a static rest state, at which all being is virtual, not manifest, which they call the *Body Without Organs*, and at which the body is free of parasitic effect of the organs.[16] Ashbery begins "The Skaters" by turning the machines into qualities of sound, as would be appropriate in the medium of language:

These decibels
Are a kind of flagellation, an entity of sound
Into which being enters, and is apart.

The sound of "these swift blades o'er the ice," from a later stanza, is like the words that fall upon the page, marking its virgin snow, as well as the poet's mind, whose thinking disrupts his peace. He has fallen from his state of grace (the *virtual*, or *static* state) into the world of the *organs*, of desire and conflict:

We children are ashamed of our bodies
But we laugh and, demanded, talk of sex again
And all is well. The waves of morning harshness
Float away like coal-gas into the sky.
But how much survives? How much of any one of us survives?

The body is *ashamed* of itself due to the work of the organs, those that *laugh*, and *talk of sex*, after passing through a difficult transition: "The waves of morning harshness. . . ." Another stable state is reached, but he asks, "How much survives? How much of any one of us survives?" But something does survive the onslaught, and in fact one learns to thrive on it and identify oneself with it:

True, Melodious tolling does go on in that awful pandemonium,
Certain resonances are not utterly displeasing to the terrified eardrum.
Some paroxysms are dinning of tamborine, others suggest piano room
    or organ loft
For the most dissonant night charms us, even after death. This, after all,
    may be happiness: tuba notes awash on the great flood, ruptures of
    xylophone, violins, limpets, grace-notes, the musical instrument
    called serpent, viola da gambas, aeolian harps, clavicles, pinball
    machines, electric drills, *que sais-je encore!*

And so the machines have their way, creating their *awful pandemonium*, their *ruptures*, and *notes awash on the great flood*. But we are charmed by the *dissonant night*. We may disappear into it for a while, or indefinitely–*The passage sustains, does not give*–yet something keeps drawing one's attention nostalgically back to the more ideal state: "And I have a dim intuition that I am that other 'I' with which we began."

This cacophony of sounds are the organs, or the desiring-machines, having their way with the *Body Without Organs,* what he senses is his original, untrammeled self, toward which he pays "A child's devotion/To this normal, shapeless entity. . . ." But whether he's willing to accept it at first, or not, he must come to terms with the fact that he is all of these voices and processes, that they are ripples on the surface of the original body. It doesn't matter if he puts up a *"No skating"* sign. The whole poem may be this *child's devotion* to a pure state of being; every scene may be "a scene worthy of the poet's pen, yet it is the fire demon/Who has created it." All the images pour out with the gas bubbles and smoke of a staged experiment, which in itself creates a separate being, springing forth others.

Ashbery's writing process is largely the content of his writing. Though he may not always know what the purpose or goal of this process might be, he is highly sensitive to what inhabits it. Just as the *body* of Deleuze and Guattari is populated by *organs*, Ashbery's inner world contains numerous mechanisms and machinations which embody his conscious process, his self or personality. Though this may be true for people in general, what makes him different is that he is attentive to them, granting them more than the usual amount of significance, allowing these internal phenomena being of their own. While a poet like Wallace Stevens may have imagined a blackbird, he may not have seen it as a manifestation of himself the way Ashbery probably would, but as a creation of his poetic imagination. The *decibels* which are *a kind of flagellation*, as well as the chorus of musical instruments, are disruptions which continually set the poem running, at one point making it come to boil, and become a "fire on the surface of the effervescent liquid," or once again: the "fire demon/Who has created" many of the scenes in part two. This is not composition in the usual sense, where the domineering ego takes the reigns and forges out a vision willfully, but more of a collaboration of a number of selves. Ashbery hears voices, not as actual hallucinations as a schizophrenic might, but through the medium of a recognizable whole, although not the unity of the typical lyrical poet. His willingness to hear himself as multiple rather than unified is what allows him to create such a vivid feeling of space in his poems, as well the sense wave.

This type of willed dissociation and objectification of the parts of oneself is not the same as, but similar to certain types of schizophrenic thinking. Someone experiencing paranoid symptoms may imagine he is hearing the voice of god, or the devil, when it is actually a part of himself he struggles to disown, and may actually carry on conversations with several imaginary personalities at once. The paranoid will *believe* these are separate entities, while Ashbery will most presumably *make believe*, as a child will when he plays with his toys. The type of thinking involved in both cases has to do with an intensified reliance on *primary function* cognition, or concretization, which corresponds with a tendency toward *fragmentation* (or *awholism*), as well as what may be called *paleological* thinking.[17]

The danger of concrete thinking is that one forgets one is thinking in metaphor, and so believes another is actually poisoning his or her food, as I mentioned before. Fragmentation usually refers to a schizophrenic's inability to visually perceive an object as a whole. For instance, he may be able to see someone's eyes, ears, mouth, and nose, but not a face. Though the mind makes an effort to construct the whole, it generally falls together in a bizarre way.

Paleologic is association by predicate, rather than subject. An example of this would be a woman believing she is the Virgin Mary because she is also a virgin: Mary was a virgin; I am a virgin; therefore I am the Virgin Mary. All three of these qualities have their equivalents in modern art, in general, but apply especially to a particular type of writing driven more by a desire to activate the power of language, than to use it merely to carry ideas across. It also represents a perspective of human existence, and its relationship to language, which has been largely overlooked by the mainstream.

As the focus of artistic endeavor has shifted from product to process, it has increasingly become the chosen task of artists to catch the mind doing what it does when it creates, or to catch language in the process of unfolding itself. This interest in the *mind in action* is not anything new, but has become a principal subject matter, since the sciences of perception and cognition have become more sophisticated, and it is found that something like the structure of language determines reality more often than reality determines it. While language used to be looked at as a neutral and objective tool to articulate a world outside of itself, it is now unreasonable to see it as such, as well as to consider there being a world we can think about outside its reach.[18] So questions like, *how does my language affect my knowing?* or *what would happen to reality if I changed the way I used language?* lose their absurdity and become the fundamental questions some poets ask throughout their careers. There have been various experiments in fragmentation done in order to approach these questions. Though some modernist and postmodernist poetry may sound like the word-salad writing of schizophrenics, it grew more out of an application of the types of things visual artists were doing, from the pointillist methods of impressionist painters, to the angular reassembly of visual space by the Picasso and Bracque. Writers like William Carlos Williams and Gertrude Stein borrowed many of their ideas from Cubism, translating the breaking down of image metaphorically into textual devices. Experiments by groups such as the French Surrealists grew out of a similar path. It made sense to ask if the known world was largely made of talk, what happened if one began to talk differently? Said in such a way, it begins to sound as though literature was trying to become a branch of science, or at least philosophy, but remember that the main initiative for seeing and saying things anew was a dissatisfaction with how things were already said and seen, and a *desire* to break new ground, to find new means of satisfaction. New York School poets, such as Ashbery and Koch, borrowing ideas from Stein and the Surrealists alike, set out to explore new ground out of the sheer fun and pleasure of doing so, believing in their hearts there was no contradiction between that and the *serious* pursuit of art.[19] Again, they found inspiration and models of fragmentation in the work of the Abstract Expressionists, which they wished to emulate in their own ways. From Stein, and the Abstract Expressionists as well, they learned that art did not have to represent nature, detached and apart from it, but that the artifact could be looked at as another aspect of life.

But what do we mean by fragmentation, and how exactly does it relate to both poetry and schizophrenia? Do we mean that the splintered schizophrenic mind is somehow closer to the primitive and unsocialized beast, Rousseau's natural man running around the forest with a more intact personal integrity and untrammeled honesty? Not quite. It's often hard to tell whether one is rediscovering forgotten ways of thinking, or inventing new ones. In most cases both are involved. As we discover that we, and the universe we live in, are less orderly and more chaotic than we had thought, it would only make sense that we would become more attracted to creative work which is in tune with that. Schizophrenia becomes a metaphor, more than a diagnosis, and the fact that we find similarities between what is usually considered a most debilitating mental illness, and some of our most interesting and healthiest of creative pursuits, is perhaps a happy sign for the well and ill alike. That is why Deleuze and Guattari exchange Freud's model of the human being as neurotic, for what they call *a schizophrenic out for a walk*, not a debilitated mental patient, but someone integrated differently, not shut down to a single, unitary *I*, or central theme, but with access to innumerable modes of being and expression. As we have seen in our discussion of Ashbery, the language we use can often carry more meaning when it isn't held to an orderly procession of reasonable gestures and assertions, but can often make an entirely more expansive statement through fragmentation and the intertwining of voices. The best poetry has always been that which has done several things at once, blending mixed or ambiguous metaphors and complex voices utilizing many forms of prosody and diction. In some contemporary poems these elements are simply more pronounced, purposely crossing the line toward a type of work that can no longer be described as making sense, or having a single voice, or purpose, in the usual sense.

Michael Palmer is another poet whose masterly use of disruption and polyvocality helps to create fragile worlds of high vibratory resonance. While often associated with language poetry, his work typically breaks free of those limits into its own form of philosophical investigation, sometimes into treatment of language and ideas reminiscent of Wittgenstein, although much more tactile and musical. There are points in which he almost seems to pull language free of the objects and events it's referencing, thereby breaking the grammatical hold, the spell with which it holds us and contextualizes everything we do and come in contact with. Whether or not this is simply illusory, he is successful enough at times to create the sensation that the thing in question has been stripped of its words, or as he puts it in "Letter 1" of "Letters to Zanzotto," where he reverses the usual naming process, by referring back to word, to language in general, with things it names:

> Wasn't it done then undone, by
> us and to us, enveloped, sid-
> erated in a starship, listing
> with liquids, helpless letters–
> what else–pouring from that box,
> little gaps, rattles and slants
>
> Like mountains, pretty much worn down
> Another sigh of breakage, wintering
> lights, towers and a century of hair,
> cloth in heaps or mounds, and limbs,
> real and artificial, to sift among[20]

These convulsing fragments break, crackle and spill over, as if from the coat of a shoplifter fleeing the scene of the crime–language describing itself "listing/with liquids," or "Like mountains pretty much worn down . . ." consisting of ". . . little gaps, rattles and slants," which are "pouring from that box." What *box* are we talking about here? *That* box, any box, which may be one of a number of mythological boxes, perhaps Pandora's, for example. While not quite personifying words and figures, Palmer refers to language with the same qualities it has granted things throughout history, and the mythic stuff in which it took root, with a schizophrenic metonymy and reversal much like primary function confusion. This is not simple metaphor, but a tearing apart of the signs in order to restore their immanence.

A more elaborate example of use of fragmentation is at use in "Sun," the first and longer poem of the same title, from the book of the same name. Here the sense of confusion and disruption extend that of the previous (although later) poem into a complex polyvocality. In this sense it almost seems to follow Ashbery's "How Much Longer . . . " in its constant dislocations and changes of direction, almost to the point of incomprehensibility. The sense that can be made from this poem cannot be gotten at by more familiar reading strategies, but by listening to how the rhythm of fragments fall, displace and punctuate each other. Take the first several lines:

> A headless man walks, lives
> for four hours
>
> devours himself
> You bring death into your mouth–X
>
> we are called–
> sleep, festinate, haul rocks[21]

The first three lines work together as a single thought: the man who survives for three hours without his head ends up devouring himself. The fourth line relates through the theme of death and *devour*ing, although the subject is no longer that of someone anonymous passing into non-being, but *you*, perhaps the speaker speaking to himself, or even the reader, who is now identified with the dead man for *bringing death into* his *mouth*. The X that follows the dash may be identified with the *death*, *you*, the *mouth*, and the *we* of the next line, which is both being called X, and being *called* to perform some action: "sleep, festinate, haul rocks." The ambiguities of identity and shifting of points of view are not merely arbitrary, or there to confuse the reader, but to exhibit the complex relationships among things in language, and how it relates to the world. In a dream state, for instance, the dreamer would be represented by all the persons, objects, and actions. Palmer is perhaps suggesting that the same thing occurs in a waking state, particularly in the act of writing and speaking. It is schizophrenic, in a sense, but at the same time the opposite is true. It is an attempt to create a hyper-lucid awareness of the way language works, or often fails to work, when connecting ideas, actions, and objects. No longer are we dealing with linear strings where one verb operates one noun, but in a constellation which grows ever more complex as the poem progresses.

As one challenges his or her sense of self or subjectivity, identifying less with the unitary "I" and more with the multiple, one can expect the same kinds of apprehensions one experiences on the analyst's couch. The ego wants to believe in its own integrity, and will at times go to war with itself in order to create boundaries where perhaps none can exist. We are "comfortable" with things because we have domesticated them, or colonized them with language, a personal adaptation of a *conventional* range of significance. I "know" what my hands are because I have been taught how to count *piggies* on them, and how to use them to eat, play, and take care of myself. My hands have meaning. But just as a word repeated over and over in the mind may be transformed into a ludicrous sound, my hand may grow unfamiliar, possibly even frightening or *awe*-inducing, when I stare at it long enough to let its physical presence overshadow its signification. A similar thing happens when one listens, by writing, to the organism which processes the language, rather than assuming a fixed role. And losing self-definition, the armor of the ego invites the anarchy of the *real*, if not to burst through the surface, at least to trace its way back and forth just below, like a shark. It makes one wonder whether true "stage fright" is really anxiety over adequately constructing and playing out a role for an audience, or in discovering that the actor and stage don't really exist, and that one is being watched by an outside and inside which are in many ways indistinguishable.

Such a perspective makes one aware of the *performance anxiety* that goes on continually in life, in every aspect, since being human involves an unrelenting struggle of self-composition. The same drives which render one whole also serve to disrupt that wholeness; the forces modeling a "self" also play a part in disintegrating it. It is of course necessary that the subject never allow itself to reach an unalterably fixed state, since it must continually adapt to the passage of time and the changing scene. The more flexible, the freer the subject, and more open to a wider range of experience, from dread to wonder, by overwriting the world with new connections and possibilities. How much is enough, too little, or too much? How can one know without exploring one's own fragmentation and schizophrenia, that journey into which possibly all journeys lead: that core adventure?

Next, in Michael Palmer's poem, we come to:

> The eye follows itself across the screen
> Words pass backward
>
> onto the tongue
> are swallows
>
> in clay cliffs
> The sea's no picture at all
>
> Blue mountain incised with a face
> ends in burnt cluster
>
> mud, private telematics, each
> person controlling a machine
>
> This is owned by the Man Roy works for
> in Insurance work
>
> Words will say this
> resolved to write a play

We are out of the mythic space of the first six lines, where headless men walk around of their own volition, and people are called on to *haul rocks*. We are suddenly behind a computer terminal, as an "eye follows itself across the screen," and "Words pass backward." There is an evolution of some sort. In the previous section, the word *sleep* is followed by another that is merely its opposite–*festinate*–which means to quicken, or enliven. This quickening eventuates a new world, much like the ordinary world we live in today, but something is equally as strange as the appearance of the "headless man" in the first line. How is it that the eye follows itself across the screen? It could be the reflection of itself it sees on the surface of the glass, but most likely not. The *eye* is intrinsically connected to the *I*, or the gaze, with which it objectifies itself, and in turn makes itself an *eye*. This is further suggested in the second line, in which "Words pass backward," reversing the order of things.

This reversal of time and causality continues into the next stanza, since the words pass backward "onto the tongue," and "are swallows." The pun on *eating one's words* is then disrupted by the associate link between the swallows of the esophagus, and the swallows that are birds, who Palmer has occupying *clay cliffs*. The *clay cliffs* are therefore associated with the tongue, and the tongue, which overlooks a "sea" which "is no picture at all," replaces the *eye*. In fact the whole mountain, which includes the cliffs, is made into a head, "incised with a face." The earth allusions rapidly turn back to technology: "ends in a burnt cluster // mud, private telematics, each/person controlling a machine."

The rest of the poem proceeds much the same way, through shards of philosophical propositions, dreamlike narratives, literary and personal anecdotes. It is inhabited by historical personages and cartoon characters who make cameo appearances for a line or two and disappear. Quite a bit of absurd attempts at naming take place, for instance: "Let's call this The Quiet City/where screams are felt as waves," and "Day One is called Tongues // Day Two might be called This-and-Only-This // Day Three is Antimony," or "Once your name was Therefore // then Rubble then Ash." The primal process of naming has therefore gone haywire: signifiers scatter and wing about like drunken birds unable to find their nests. In Yeats's words, "The center cannot hold," and without the much relied-on system of articulation intact the landscape falls back into a primordial ooze. Language in the meantime is having itself quite a party, kind of a costume ball, in which terms dress up as one another, but still contain at center a holograph of the thing it had left behind. The effect on the reader, once he or she has gotten the gist, may be something similar to a vacation in a foreign land with a drastically different culture, so that some of the novelty and disorientation remains on returning home.

NOTES

1. Friedrich Nietzsche, *The Gay Science.* Trans. Walter Kaufman.

2. David Lehman, *The Last Avant-Garde: the making of the New York School of Poets.* New York: Doubleday, 1998. "I am nature," says Jackson Pollock.

3. Silvano Altieri, *Interpretation of Schizophrenia.* New York: Basic Books, 1974.

4. ibid.

5. ibid.

6. Gilles Deleuze, Felix Guattari, *Anti-Oedipus: Capitalism and Schizophrenia.* Trans. Robert Hurley, Mark Seem, and Helen R. Lane. Minneapolis: University of Minnesota Press, 1983. Gilles Deleuze, Felix Guattari, *A Thousand Plateaus.* Trans. Brian Massumi. Minneapolis: University of Minnesota Press, 1987.

7. John Ashbery, *The Tennis Court Oath.* Reprinted as part of *The Mooring of Starting Out.* New York: The Ecco Press, 1997.

8. Jacques Lacan, *The Four Fundamental Concepts of Psychoanalysis*, Ed. Jacques-Alain Miller, Trans. Alan Sheridan, New York and London, W. W. Norton & Company, 1977.

9. Bob Perelman, *The Marginalization of Poetry: Language Writing and Literary History.* Princeton: Princeton University Press, 1996.

10. *Everybody's Autobiography.* Gertrude Stein. Cambridge: Exact Change, 1993.

11. Perelman.

12. *Language poets* approach language as their primary subject matter.

13. Since Freud we have all become layman analysts and self-analysts.

14. *A User's Guide to Capitalism and Schizophrenia.* Brian Massumi. Cambridge: A Swerve Addition, MIT Press, 1992.

15. ibid.

16. It is here that they owe much to the writings of Artaud.

17. Arieti.

18. *Wittgenstein's Ladder*, Marjorie Perloff. Chicago and London: University of Chicago Press, 1996.

19. Lehman.

20. Michael Palmer, *At Passages.* New York: New Directions, 1995.

21. Michael Palmer, *Sun.* San Francisco: North Point Press, 1988.

In Awe of the Superindividual:
A Conversation with E. Mark Stern
and Rob Marchesani

RM: In your article "The Awesome and the Awestruck" you describe what clinicians might see in patients who suffer in their attachments. There is a kind of awe that is blinding and even denigrating to the beholder. "He is everything; I am nothing," might be the subtext of one who stands in awe of another. That may further develop into: "With him I am everything; without him I am nothing." Does this kind of awe come with an idealization? Or is it something else?

EMS: Idealization is one way of pacing values. Heroes are idealized. They foster personal nourishment. We idealize another as a standard for what may or may not be our own possibility. Idolization is quite another process. The idolizer is disjointed. He or she declares a sense of worthlessness. An idol represents the only "hope" for a real existence. In a short story by Tennessee Williams, "The Black Masseur," a white patron of a health club makes arrangements for a series of intense rubdowns by a super-strong black masseur. Over a period of time, the massages get violent. The patron begins to

---

E. Mark Stern, EdD, ABPP (Diplomate in Clinical Psychology), is a Fellow of the American Psychological Association, the American Psychological Society, and the Academy of Clinical Psychology. He is Emeritus Professor, Graduate School of Arts and Sciences at Iona College in New Rochelle, NY. Dr. Stern is in private practice of psychotherapy in New York City and Clinton Corners in Dutchess County, NY.

Rob Marchesani is a psychotherapist in private practice in New York City where he teaches "The Internet and the Hyper-Self" at The New School in Greenwich Village. In 1996 he appeared in the Beth B film *Visiting Desire,* a documentary on fantasy and sexual relations which entered the Toronto and Berlin film festivals after playing at Cinema Village. He holds a Masters from The New School and is co-editor of *The Psychotherapy Patient* series.

[Haworth co-indexing entry note]: "In Awe of the Superindividual: A Conversation with E. Mark Stern and Rob Marchesani." Stern, E. Mark, and Rob Marchesani. Co-published simultaneously in *The Psychotherapy Patient* (The Haworth Press, Inc.) Vol. 11, No. 3/4, 2001, pp. 223-228; and: *Frightful Stages: From the Primitive to the Therapeutic* (ed: Robert B. Marchesani, and E. Mark Stern) The Haworth Press, Inc., 2001, pp. 223-228. Single or multiple copies of this article are available for a fee from The Haworth Document Delivery Service [1-800-342-9678, 9:00 a.m. - 5:00 p.m. (EST). E-mail address: getinfo@haworthpressinc.com].

sport stark bruises and broken limbs. The proprietor of the gym expels both of them. The "couple" rent a small apartment in a run-down New Orleans neighborhood. There the "massage" continues on and on with more shattered limbs. Eventually the masseur cannibalizes his patron. Williams was edging on the danger of idolatry. The masseur is made to play the subterraneous object of worship while his devotee is left with no sense of existence. The "solution" is to be animated–made alive, by being incorporated in the body of the victim-nourished "god."

RM: That's interesting and may be more applicable today than when Williams wrote the story. There seem to be more body crazes in a kind of worshipful way. Gyms, personal trainers, home exercise machines all seem as though they are helping the person develop into something better. But I wonder about the fact that heroes, and I mean the ones we see from the time we are children–everyone from Batman and Superman to nearly all the Marvel Comics' masters, even the plastic toys and dolls, all have great physiques bordering on the grotesque. At the New Museum of Contemporary Art's exhibition (March 30-June 25, 2000), "Picturing the Modern Amazon" sported the physique of a hypermuscular black woman subtitled: "curiously strong women," a pun on the Altoids ad which sponsored the exhibition.[1] What's this do to the poor flabby kid? What's this do to the skinny kid? Eating disorders are another manifestation of this body craze gone crazy. And it occurs in men as well. But I'm also thinking of the other heroes, those people we call stars, whether Broadway, Hollywood, or those of the sports arenas. Is there a kind of idolatry of stardom that denigrates the ordinary? One that diminishes the person in the darkness of the audience or at home disconnected by the distance from the reality behind the tube or in the magazine?

EMS: Heroes call forth admiration. The mythic hero inspires not only a generation but an entire culture. Then there are the personal heroes. Especially in children, the enhanced hero may be a role model. I recall once reading about a child who donned his new Superman costume and hurled himself out of a six-story building with the intention of soaring in the air as his hero Superman.

I once worked with a man who was "addicted" to photographing high school football heroes. They were the gods of his sheltered basement. Glaring at the vanishing athlete in full regalia enabled his fantasies to transform him into the bodies of those he awed. Through one orifice or another, he'd "enter" into the boy hero's torso. In his fantasy, he would then spread his arms, creep into the boy's arms, allow his legs to pierce the boy's legs, his head to complete the idol. In the end, he'd don the shoulder pads and helmet of a football player.

Mircea Eliade might refer to such fantasies as existing in "profane time," a way of enlisting the hero to unleash those who are terrified from the terror of their ordinary reality.

Recall Jeffrey Dahmer. He seduced and murdered countless numbers of young men. He would preserve his victim's body as long as he could; share his bed with the dead body, and as a final meshing, resorted to cannibalization. This drive toward inclusion became his desperate attempt at remediating the experience of nonbeing. Stalking a rejecting "idol" is much along this same pathway.

RM: It seems to me that these darker sides of awe are occurring within psychotic and perverse structures. The more neurotic may have less severe outcomes or at least less extreme, but perhaps as tragic, at least where the awestruck doesn't resituate her or his relationship with the object of awe. The dark side of awe seems like a kind of getting off, nonsexual turn-on, though in some cases they are indeed sexualized as in the ones you just described. I dare say that the ritual of the Mass includes a similar kind of awe which follows another kind of consumption of an idealized as well as idolized body and soul of the Christ figure. No doubt the artists of generations have unconsciously painted this Christ with his "six pack" abs and sinewy naked body displayed for all on which to lock their gaze. A figure of purity that has captured the imagination and desire of millions. It is a frozen image. Awe seems to border on a kind of hysteria which captures men and women alike. There is a photo of a concert with Paul McCartney which struck me as speaking to this. It was on the cover of a magazine. In this crowd were the most pained faces of young women who seemed tortured by their overwhelming desire for this man, if it was that. He'd become an icon for them but one which clearly diminished them as it aggrandized him.

EMS: So awe is enrapturing, holding its objects in a paralyzing head lock. But is it sex? Most certainly there are sexual overtones. My sense is that awe which idolizes is the state of not-being-alive-in-myself. Being thus awed is the flawed attempt to come alive in the consumption of the idol. Cult adherents view their leaders, not as heroes, but as idols who contain them. An icon, on the other hand, can either be an object of adulation or a way to the sacred mysteries of existence. Mystical experience is yet another kettle of fish.

William James identified the mystical experience as the embodiment of four qualities: ineffability, which, by inference, resembles negative awe, seeking being in non-being. James's second property of mysticism is the noetic. In this state individuals enlarge personal awareness. Transiency suggests that mystical awareness is like an escaping dream. And finally, passivity sequences spectatorship into surrender. Despite fleetingness and surrender, what is truly mystical is never actually lost to the moment, but rather engaged by it.

Awe, in its terror, is neither aesthetic nor enlarging. Those so seized cease to claim their being. A man I once worked with in therapy was unusually prone to accidents. On the day he scheduled an initial consultation with me, he was hit by a speeding bicycle and had to be rushed to a hospital emergency room. This was only one in a series of such incidents. So out of touch with his aliveness that he paid prostitutes to lock him in a dark closet for 48 hours at a time. He fantasized his "captor" as a strong, but rejecting, mother. His hell was the ever-present revivification of his tormented infancy. It may be one thing to adulate a fetish, and quite another to be supplanted by a devouring other. Some are devoured by their work, others overwhelmed by obsession. There are people so engulfed by the overflowing dam of unconsciousness (spiked narcotic episodes). These states are all akin to the stupefaction of an unrelenting awe.

RM: In a short interview with Martin Scorcese about his films, he said that there were feelings he might not have been ready to verbalize that came out in his pictures. I think what Freud was after with the unconscious was to take those raw pictures and put words to them. Yet, artists seem to love the pictures first–the raw feelings that enrapture. The garden had to be created before it was named, or so the story is told. Which makes one wonder if there is a place for making things before knowing what they are. It may be enough to know *that* they are before the naming occurs. I wonder, in our work with patients, if this is not the place of observation before rushing in to say what's going on. To let sleeping dogs lie so they can have their dream before the rational comes in.

EMS: I agree. Sleeping dogs ought to be allowed to sleep. But never forget even the sleeping dog is busy with REM dreaming. Dreaming is often unrecognized awe.

RM: So, can awe be a kind of denial? Or is it one of many inescapable human experiences of oneself and another?

EMS: Awe, at its deepest, is the terror of the overpowering, overarching other demanding a relinquishment of all power. But at its best awe may lure the individual in to an enlargement of self precisely because of the surrender to a greater other. That "greater" other may literally be *an* other person, or it may be *an* overwhelming event, a realization of the unbounded cosmos. Awe is not a defense in the usual psychodynamic sense.

On a positive note, the awed may be "glorified" by ingesting a greater entity, such as the Eucharist, the heart of a felled hero, or by the deep identification with an object of aesthetic appeal or desire.

RM: I've certainly fallen in awe of someone. That sounds strange but it isn't so strange. Awe is a kind of infatuation, on one level. On another level, it becomes something deeper, more profound. I've been in awe of people I imagined to be great in some way or in all ways without differentiating the ways. When the time to differentiate the ways comes, the awe sometimes subsides. But I must say the best remedy for awe, at its worst, is a healthy boost in oneself, in one's worth. I think when two people become in awe of something they share that's greater than each of them, then there can be a profound transformation.

EMS: Perhaps awe should have no remedy since it provides a personal vantage point. Awe bypasses and goes around the ego. In its action, awe renames ego, not as superego, but as superindividuality.

RM: How so?

EMS: Superindividuality was a term first applied to personality theory by Andras Angyal. Superindividuality happens when two or more autonomies create a third possibility. Superindividuality, as I use the term, suggests the most positive dimensions of awe. Individuality is transcended even as autonomy is enlarged. For an infinite second or for a codified lifetime the whole is transformed–not enraptured. The affective state of awe is a convergence of wonder and dread.

RM: Art seems to be a call to life, or to the hidden in life. Art opens the heart, suggests Jeannette Winterson (1995) in *Art Objects: Essays on Ecstasy and Effrontery,* who states that art doesn't imitate life as much as it anticipates life. She concludes that the artist imagines the forbidden because to her it is not forbidden. Art seems to be an integral part of many a psychotherapist's office. Whether noticed or not, it seems to have colored the walls and surfaces of such chambers since Freud first talked to the sculptures that still sit on his desk in his study at Marsfield Gardens in London long after his death. Art seems to call us into and out of those most personal spaces and places of contemplation, like the mirror which the artist turns into a self-portrait for the eyes of others. After I brought a piece of sculpture into my office, a patient, after many private contemplations, turned to it and said, "That's exactly how I feel!" She also said it in another session when she stood and turned to look at a painting above the couch. So art seems to encompass emotions which sometimes remain inarticulable until they are seen, framed by a form.

EMS: Anticipation, whether of art or sex, is both terrifying and exciting. Is awe always anticipating something beyond itself? Is awe the great trickster? Disappointment often follows, except in those instances where anticipation awakens awe.

Awe is a unitive experience either in anticipation or in the moment. Some who are attracted to ardent self-denial may see it as a path leading to a oneness with something or somebody beyond themselves: an integration of self with non-self.

Eastern religion and Western mysticism key in on the dissolution of self. Awe, for such movements, provides a total vantage point. If I be nothing, then it follows that I am all. But with idolization, something else takes place. Awe is not about seeking unity. It is more that one has never existed before.

RM: Just this morning I stood outside the doors of the church of my childhood along with a friend I'd met in that church's school. The service for his mother's funeral was over. There was a box on the steps which I noticed when I stepped off the last and onto the sidewalk. A man took the box, opened the top and slid back the wooden lid. There the head of a white dove appeared. He took the bird in his hands and placed it in my friend's who held onto it with one hand while he held his youngest daughter of one and a half in his other arm. He waited until she reached out and placed her hand on the feathered creature. The man took the basket and said that it was our friend's wish to release these three doves in honor of his mother who so loved birds. This friend and the man stood waiting to open the box to release the other two and to let go of the one in his hand. He looked up, raised his hand and opened it with a look of some kind of pain and separation I'd never seen in a person's face. The three doves flew together over our heads and into the blue cloudless morning sky until they disappeared over the houses.

EMS: What incredible imagery. You highlight an awe, fully realized and available: an essential of aesthetic freedom. It is also wise to resist the lures of awe. Recall Plato's advice that it is best to relinquish the dovishness of tranquility in favor of the pandemonium of day-to-day life in the ordinary world. So awe leaves off as utopia or hell, depending on context.

NOTE

1. The exhibition "features over a century of images, exploring the fascinating phenomenon of the hypermuscular woman and her role in popular culture and contemporary art."

Index

8 1/2 (F. Fellini), 77,90

Abbey of Gethsemani (Kentucky), 38,
    45-46
Abraham (Biblical character), xiii-xiv
Abraham, K., 47
Action therapies, 99-121
Adler, E., 112
Ahern, B.A., 48
Alexander, F., 43
Alexander, T. (pseud.), 181-185
Altered states, 181-185
American, 29
American Academy of
    Psychotherapists, 115-116
American Psychological Association
    (APA), 7,164
Angel, E., 137-140
Anguish and awe
    introduction to, 169-170
    personal experience case studies,
        170-180
    research about, 180
Anxiety (E. Munch), 2-3
APA. *See* American Psychological
    Association (APA)
Apollonian awe, xiii-xiv, 99-121
Aprile, D., 46,53
Aristotle, 3
Armstrong, L., 74
Arpesella, P., 6,197-203
*Art Objects: Essays on Ecstasy and
    Effrontery* (J. Winterson), 227
Art of the Obvious, The (B.
    Bettelheim and A.
    Rosenfeld), 96-97
Artistic creation
    awe, introduction to, 1-9. *See also*
        Awe

Harlem Renaissance, 27-35
poetic schizophrenia and awe,
    205-221
spontaneity and, 1-9
stage fright and. *See* Stage fright
Artistic works
    Anxiety (E. Munch), 2-3
    God Mother, 56
    musical. *See* Musical works
    Scream (E. Munch), 2-3
Ashbery, J., 205-221
Augustine (Saint), xiii-xiv, 7-8,25
Awe
    action therapies and, 99-121
    altered states and, 181-185
    anguish and, 169-180
    Apollonian, xiii-xiv, 99-121
    artistic creation and, 1-9
    awestruck persons and, 27-35
    definition of, xiii-xiv, 126
    Dionysian, xiii-xiv, 99-121
    experiential personal construct
        psychology and, 123-127,
        149-162
    experiential sessions and, 129-147
    idealization and idolization,
        223-228
    importance of, 163-167
    insight and expression, polarity
        between, 99-121
    introduction to, xiii-xiv, 1-9,
        123-124
    mystery and, 163-167
    narcissism and, 12
    normality and, 125-126
    poetic schizophrenia and, 205-221
    psychotherapeutic healing and,
        123-127
    research about, 127,167,228
    reverence and, 149-162. *See also*

For Product Safety Concerns and Information please contact our EU representative GPSR@taylorandfrancis.com Taylor & Francis Verlag GmbH, Kaufingerstraße 24, 80331 München, Germany

T - #0039 - 160425 - C0 - 229/152/13 [15] - CB - 9780789013651 - Gloss Lamination